BORDERLINE DISORDERS
Clinical Models and Techniques

BORDERLINE DISORDERS

Clinical Models and Techniques

EDA G. GOLDSTEIN

THE GUILFORD PRESS
New York   London

To Dr. Marjorie Taggart White

A courageous pioneer and an optimally responsive selfobject

© 1990 The Guilford Press
A Division of Guilford Publications, Inc.
72 Spring Street, New York, NY 10012

Printed in the United States of America

This book is printed on acid-free paper.

Last digit is print number: 9   8   7   6   5   4   3   2   1

Library of Congress Cataloging-in-Publication Data

Goldstein, Eda G.
　　Borderline disorders : clinical models and techniques / Eda G. Goldstein.
　　　　p.　cm.
　　Includes bibliographical references.
　　Includes index.
　　ISBN 0-89862-442-8
　　1. Borderline personality disorder.　　I. Title.
　　[DNLM: 1. Borderline Personality Disorder.　　WM 190 G6237b]
RC569.5.B67G65　　1990
616.85'852 — dc20
DNLM/DLC
for Library of Congress　　　　　　　　　　　　　　　　90-3400
　　　　　　　　　　　　　　　　　　　　　　　　　　　　　　CIP

Acknowledgments

I have been very fortunate to have worked closely with two individuals who have contributed greatly to the development of different approaches to the diagnosis and treatment of patients with narcissistic and borderline pathology. After just completing my doctoral studies at the Columbia University School of Social Work in 1973, my 7-year collaboration with Dr. Otto Kernberg began. While not sharing his views, I shall always be grateful for his confidence in my abilities and for the opportunity he gave me to be so closely involved with the evolution, teaching, and research of his ego psychological–object relations approach to borderline disorders. Numerous colleagues in the Borderline Research Group, which Dr. Kernberg and I co-led both at the New York State Psychiatric Institute and at the New York Hospital–Cornell Medical Center, Westchester Division, provided me with an intellectually dynamic environment. Later, when I became more immersed in self psychology, I benefited considerably from my association with Dr. Marjorie Taggart White and many members of her seminar, Self Psychology for Practicing Psychotherapists. I shall be forever thankful to Dr. White for her vision and example and for the lively discussions in which we thrashed out many of the vexing issues with which one is confronted in the self psychological treatment of individuals with severe developmental arrests.

Dean Shirley Ehrenkranz, Associate Dean Eleanor Korman, Dr. George Frank, Dr. Burt Shacter, Dr. Judith Mishne, Dr. Jeffrey Seinfeld, and Dr. Judith Siegel of the New York University School of Social Work have all been important sources of support and collegiality. The School has been extremely hospitable to my work and professional interests over the past 9 years. To the numerous hospital and social work agency staffs that I have spoken to about borderline and narcissistic disorders in recent times, I must say a special thanks for their interest in and response to my ideas.

Two friends, Dr. Lucille Spira and Dr. Jill Morris, have listened patiently and offered their excellent ideas during the period in which I have been preparing this manuscript. Ms. Pat Petrocelli also has been a staunch supporter. Ms. Sharon Panulla of Guilford Press has been all that a fine editor should be. Mr. Richard Lenert has provided me with invaluable secretarial and administrative assistance. Lastly, I am grateful to my students, supervisees, and patients who have been a constant source of inspiration and renewal.

Contents

PART I

HISTORICAL DEVELOPMENTS AND CURRENT PERSPECTIVES

1

Introduction: The Challenge of the Borderline Patient

In recent years mental health clinicians have shown an avid interest in the study of borderline disorders. Practitioners of many disciplines in psychiatric hospitals and clinics, health and social agencies, and private practice frequently encounter many so-called borderline individuals in their work, but often are baffled, drained, and frustrated by the tumultuous and unrelenting nature of their particular problems. Consequently, it is commonplace for clinicians to regard these patients as "difficult" to treat. They arouse strong emotions in the therapeutic personnel with whom they come in contact. Although these patients are frequently intelligent, talented, and appealing, their problems seriously interfere with their personal and social functioning. When involved in treatment they challenge clinicians' empathic capacities, standard repertoire of skills, and cherished beliefs about what is supposed to happen in the treatment process, and often, despite considerable treatment, their problems remain entrenched.

TURBULENT LIVES

Leading lives of not so quiet desperation, borderline individuals are often angry, volatile, impulsive, and self-destructive. Highly contradictory in their feelings and behavior, they simultaneously yearn for and are threatened by closeness with others. Plagued by fears of abandonment and riddled with separation anxiety, they often alternate between merging and distancing behavior. Many show severe identity disturbances and develop brief psychotic episodes. These patients are highly sensitive to rejection, disappointment, or criticism, and their self-esteem fluctuates dramatically. They do not tolerate stress well and often are flooded by anxiety. These characteristics show themselves in their day to day functioning, and also appear in the treatment relationship.

For example, Nancy, a 23-year-old, single recent college graduate who worked in the advertising field behaved so differently in each of her therapy sessions that it was difficult to get a sense of the "real" Nancy or to predict what she would do next. Over the course of four consecutive meetings, Nancy alternately appeared haughty and challenging, eager to please and ingratiating, depressed and self-reflective, or anxious and disorganized. The therapist was at a loss to understand what in herself or the patient provoked these changing self-presentations, which sometimes occurred within a single session. When the therapist drew attention to Nancy's shifting states and attempted to explore their meaning, Nancy abruptly changed the subject. She would frequently telephone her therapist between sessions and if the therapist attempted to set limits by telling Nancy not to call after 10 p.m., she was sure to call at 10:05 p.m. Sometimes she called within minutes of leaving the session to ask if the therapist was angry at her. On other occasions she would leave a series of messages on the therapist's answering machine during an evening: "I just want you to know how much I love you. So when are you going to call me back? Fuck you, I never want to see you again! I'm sorry—cancel all the previous messages." Upon leaving a session there were times when Nancy would announce that the therapist obviously did not care about her and that if she did not hear from Nancy again it was because she had killed herself.

CRISES IN TREATMENT

It is not easy to form or maintain therapeutic alliances with borderline patients. Even treatments with successful outcomes usually are stormy and characterized by frequent disruptions. Some of the more common difficulties that patients show include: missed appointments; threats to leave and actual withdrawal from treatment; alcohol, drug, and food abuse; self-mutilation; non-payment of fees; non-compliance with agency or therapeutic requirements; suicidal rumination and gestures; insistent requests for personal information, additional time, or extra-therapeutic contact; and behavior that requires hospitalization or elicits the therapist's active involvement in the patient's life. One of the most frustrating features of many of these disruptions is their suddenness. They seem to occur without apparent warning, although the therapist may learn that the problems have been brewing for a long time. Borderline patients often do not spontaneously discuss significant and troubling aspects of their current lives in treatment, as is shown in the following vignette.

Barbara, a 30-year-old psychiatric nurse, sought help for depression following the breakup of a highly volatile marriage. Although she was unusually vague about the details of her current life, she shared her feelings about past life experiences easily. When attempting to clarify how Barbara was presently doing at work or in her significant relationships, the therapist felt as if she was "grilling" Barbara. However, she did not explore her apparent withholding lest she appear to be accusatory. Barbara's depression lifted quickly and she reported feeling in more control of her life. Several months into the treatment, when a check with which Barbara paid her fee bounced, the therapist was dismayed to learn that Barbara's financial life was in such chaos that she was considering declaring bankruptcy. She had never made reference to her deteriorating economic circumstances. While this financial crisis was averted when Barbara's mother came to the rescue, another occurred several months later after another seemingly productive period in the treatment. This time the therapist received an angry call from Barbara's mother, who berated the therapist for being "taken in" by and not "tough enough" with Barbara, and who threatened to stop paying for Barbara's treatment. The mother informed the surprised therapist that Barbara had just been fired from her job after having received numerous warnings about her failing performance.

DERAILMENTS OF THE
THERAPEUTIC RELATIONSHIP

In the preceding example the therapist's lack of awareness of significant aspects of Barbara's life contributed to the crises in her treatment. While many clinicians believe that borderline patients commonly show distorted perceptions of the therapist, often, rigid or unattuned therapeutic interventions trigger disturbances in the treatment relationship. For example, a chronically depressed man lapsed into a noncommunicative and sullen state when his therapist erroneously interpreted his lack of zest as being a result of his identification with his depressed father. This unempathic comment made the patient feel blamed and misunderstood. His reaction worsened when the therapist suggested that the patient's silent withdrawal was evidence of his resistance to this interpretation. In another instance, an intensely lonely and desperate woman, who had been severely neglected as a child, felt her therapist's well-intentioned but persistent refusal to answer personal questions to be so depriving and so reminiscent of her isolated upbringing that she left treatment precipitously.

While therapeutic errors or insensitivity can lead to disruptions in the treatment more than is generally thought in work with borderline patients, even attuned and flexible therapists may not be able to prevent derailments of the therapeutic relationship at times. Highly charged patient reactions may be stimulated by what appears to be minor lapses in the therapist's attention or even by seemingly empathic but nevertheless threatening comments. Consequently, therapists frequently experience insecurity and the feeling that they are "walking a tightrope" in the treatment. For example, one man became angry when his therapist sneezed several times during a session. He accused the therapist of being preoccupied with himself. When the therapist somewhat incredulously indicated that he had a cold, the patient angrily accused the therapist of blaming him (the patient) for his own inadequacies, threatened to quit treatment, and stormed out of the session. In later meetings, the therapist found himself straining to pay close attention to the patient for fear that he might erupt again. In another instance, an attractive but guarded woman patient canceled a session in order to have her hair cut. This followed a session in which she tearfully expressed feeling understood and accepted by the therapist. When the patient appeared at her next appointment she spoke of her suicidal feelings after the last session and verbally attacked the therapist for being cold and indifferent. The therapist was quite dismayed. He felt that he had reacted warmly to the patient's comments, and that it was she who had distanced herself from him. After this incident the therapist became concerned about showing his feelings since he thought that he had frightened the patient.

NEGATIVE COUNTERTRANSFERENCE

While many therapists bring a high degree of commitment, if not an almost heroic effort, to the treatment of borderline individuals, there is no other patient group, with the possible exception of those who are anti-social, about whom so many negatively tinged terms are used.

Among these are manipulative, demanding, sadistic, controlling, infantile, and provocative. While at times therapists' countertransference reactions lead them to attempt to rescue these patients, often their problems are seen pejoratively rather than with empathy. Angry responses, power struggles, and therapeutic stalemates develop. Reiser and Levenson (1984) note that the use of the borderline diagnosis itself is commonly abused to express countertransference hate, to rationalize mistakes or treatment failures, or as a justification for therapist acting-out. There is a need to be ever vigilant about the host of potentially countertherapeutic reactions that borderline patients may induce or stimulate at times during treatment.

COLLABORATIVE IMPASSES

Collaborative difficulties among the members of the therapeutic team commonly accompany the treatment of borderline patients. Such divisiveness is readily apparent on in-patient psychiatric units or in other types of residential settings where staff interact closely. It is just as great a hazard in out-patient or private practice, however, where those professionals who may not even know one another but who are involved with the patient find themselves sometimes quite angry at, envious of, or even disdainful of one another. In both types of settings intense feelings or disputes can arise that might center, for example, on one staff member's view of the patient as vulnerable, needy, and requiring nurture, while another staff member views the patient as aggressive and provocative, needing clear limits and a firm therapeutic stance. Others line up on different sides of this debate, which may become highly personalized and polarized. The following vignette shows the strain that developed in the treatment of a hospitalized borderline patient among the in-patient staff and between the hospital and private therapists involved in the case.

Ellen, an attractive 25-year-old artist, was admitted to the hospital after she took an overdose of sleeping pills during her psychoanalyst's brief vacation. She was discovered by her mother who rushed her to the hospital. The psychiatric resident who was assigned to Ellen's case found her to be quite sensitive and fragile, and believed her description of her analyst as cold and punitive. As a consequence the resident did not call him. Ellen used her sessions with the resident to ventilate her anger at both her analyst and her mother, the latter of whom she called "the witch." When Ellen complained about her problems with the nursing staff, the resident was amused by her description of them as "bitter old maids" and believed that they were being too hard on her.

Feeling he was really helping Ellen, who praised him for his talent and special sensitivity, the resident felt good when he left their sessions. He was therefore shocked when he received a call early one Sunday morning from the head nurse announcing that Ellen had swallowed the sleeping pills that she been hoarding. Monday morning staff rounds revealed that Ellen had been quite stubborn and angry since her admission to the unit, often speaking abusively to the nurses. When they urged the resident to deal with Ellen's provocative behavior, he had ignored them. They became angry, and thought that Ellen was manipulating him. On the Friday before her suicidal gesture Ellen began disparaging the resident and complained to the nurses about his stupidity and insensitivity. They admitted being pleased that he was her "target" for a change. In a telephone call the resident received from Ellen's analyst, whom Ellen had contacted just prior to her most recent suicide attempt, he learned that prior to Ellen's first suicide attempt she had proclaimed her love for the analyst. He, however, was annoyed at the resident for not consulting him, and so had not initiated contact himself since he feared that the hospital would resent his intrusion.

FAMILY PATHOLOGY

Family relationships of borderline patients present their own host of difficulties and often reflect shared pathology. Couple interactions are turbulent and conflicted, and often alternate between merging and distancing behaviors. The couple has trouble living together and may frequently separate, but cannot live apart for long and reconcile. Parent–child relationships generally are characterized either by rejection or enmeshment. While maladaptive family patterns may result from the presence of a borderline member, entrenched family pathology usually aggravates or perpetuates the patient's problems. Those practitioners who work with borderline families frequently find them hard to engage collaboratively in treatment efforts. Because they often experience the relatives as demanding, hostile, intrusive, or uncaring, it is not uncommon for therapeutic personnel to find it difficult to empathize with their undermining behavior. At the same time, family members may view some staff attitudes and treatment practices as psychologically assaulting. These may escalate family members' anxiety and low self-esteem and activate seemingly pathological family responses. The following example shows a complex, family-transactional pattern. Notice both how the family stimulated the patient's problems and how certain treatment recommendations provoked the family.

Mr. and Mrs. Whiteman and their 20-year-old daughter, Susan, had consulted three psychiatrists during the past year regarding Susan's agoraphobic and depressive symptoms. She was fearful of leaving the house alone, and was dependent on the company of one or both of her parents. Each psychiatrist advised the parents that they were overprotecting and infantilizing Susan, who needed to become independent of them. They all recommended individual treatment for Susan and urged the parents to encourage her to move into a separate apartment. The family seemingly complied with the recommendations. As soon as Susan moved out, however, they barraged her with telephone calls in which they inquired about her emotional state and complained of their marital fights. Susan then demanded that her parents take her to her psychotherapy sessions as she was frightened to go alone. Soon they were accompanying her wherever she wanted to go. After becoming resentful at her constant requests for their help and angry at the psychiatrists for their recommendations, Mr. and Mrs. Whiteman prevailed upon Susan to leave treatment and move back home. At age 20 she had not worked since leaving high school or attended college, and rarely socialized with peers except on the telephone. After moving out and returning home three times, Susan became increasingly withdrawn and depressed and made the suicide attempt that led to her first psychiatric hospitalization. The Whitemans became panicky when informed by the admissions office of the unit policy of no visiting during the evaluation period, and they attempted to see her anyway. The staff had to ask them repeatedly to leave the unit. The social worker assigned to the case received daily telephone calls from the Whitemans, and her repeated reassurances that Susan was doing well did not alleviate their anxiety. They complained that Susan's therapist blamed them for her problems and demanded to see the psychiatrist in charge. When he advised them that Susan might benefit from a longer hospitalization they indicated their preference that she return home, and as a result she was soon discharged against medical advice.

DIVERGENT THEORETICAL AND
CLINICAL MODELS

What are borderline disorders? What causes this complex pathology? How should borderline conditions be treated? Since the emergence of the term "borderline" (Stern, 1938), a large and still growing literature has accumulated that attempts to answer these questions. Despite the outpouring of books and articles on this topic, however, there is considerable disagreement and controversy regarding all these issues as will be discussed in more detail in Chapter 2. For example, the most recent versions of the *Diagnostic and Statistical Manual of Mental Disorders* (DSM-III, DSM-III-R; American Psychiatric Association, 1980, 1987) classifies borderline conditions as one type of personality disorder. Kernberg (1975, 1984) differs and views borderline conditions as reflecting a pathological defensive organization that underlies many personality disorders. In contrast, Brandchaft and Stolorow (1984a, 1984b) argue that the extreme behavior that results in the diagnosis of a fixed borderline structure actually is produced by therapists' lack of empathy and unattuned therapeutic interventions. Biologically oriented theorists such as Kety, Rosenthal, Wender, and Schulsinger (1968), Akiskal (1981), and Klein (1977) do not regard borderline phenomena as constituting a distinct diagnostic category at all but rather classify them as variants of either schizophrenic or affective disorders.

A major disagreement among the psychodynamically oriented writers on borderline conditions centers on whether these conditions reflect a pathological defensive organization that wards off intrapsychic *conflict* (Kernberg, 1975, 1984; Masterson, 1972, 1976; Masterson & Rinsley, 1975) or whether they stem from a lack of internal structure and represent ego or self *deficits* (G. Blanck & R. Blanck, 1974, 1979; Buie & Adler, 1982; Adler, 1985; Kohut, 1971, 1977, 1984; Tolpin, 1980). Treatment models are divergent and contradictory. For example, the conflict-based approaches of Kernberg and Masterson are not only different from one another but are quite disparate from the various deficit-based models of G. Blanck and R. Blanck, Adler and Buie, Kohut, and others. Further, none of these approaches give a prominent role to the use of medication that is advocated by the biologically oriented clinicians (Klein, 1977) except in selected instances.

These differing theoretical and clinical models present the practitioner with a bewildering array of conflicting choices. Accounts of successfully treated borderline patients do not clarify which approach is optimal (Waldinger & Gunderson, 1987), and there are no systematic research studies that report on the outcome of different treatments with this population at the present time.

Because clinicians have tended to view borderline disorders exclusively from psychodynamic or biological perspectives, the literature on this topic, with some notable exceptions (Shapiro et al., 1975, 1977), virtually ignores family systems thinking and couple and family treatment. Yet, those who have worked on in-patient psychiatric units know that the families of borderline patients are crucial to successful treatment. Further, the vast numbers of emotionally disturbed adolescents and young adults who live with or are otherwise dependent on their families underscore the importance of family involvement in both in- and out-patient treatment. Similarly, many borderline patients are in relationships with partners who also may be borderline themselves and/or whose particular emotional problems and responses may be contributing to marital or couple discord. The treatment of borderline couples and families is an important concern of many clinicians and requires more extensive consideration than it has been given thus far.

THE BOOK'S PERSPECTIVE

For many years I have known that someday I would write a book about borderline disorders. My views on this subject, however, have changed radically over time. In 1973 I became involved in developing and coordinating a research project on the hospital treatment of borderline conditions in collaboration with Drs. Otto Kernberg, Michael Stone, and others at the New York State Psychiatric Institute. At that time I was interested in the integration of individual and family treatment in work with severely disturbed patients. In 1977, our work moved to the New York Hospital, Cornell Medical Center, Westchester Division. In both of these settings our clinical and research efforts attracted many prominent visitors, some of whom were also on the cutting edge of the study of borderline disorders. It was an exciting time as we tried to implement and study an optimal therapeutic milieu for the treatment of borderline disorders according to Kernbergian principles, and as different views were aired and hotly debated.

My clinical work with borderline patients and their families continued during this period and gradually compelled me to experiment with different therapeutic approaches. Numerous questions gnawed at me such as: Is there only one type of or a range of borderline disorders? Is borderline pathology reflective of a rigid and maladaptive defensive structure or indicative of profound and early developmental deficits? Are the confrontation and interpretation of primitive defenses and character patterns the most effective ways of helping patients or do they aggravate their difficulties, sometimes stimulating seemingly pathological responses? Should technical neutrality, as opposed to real or selfobject experiences, be the essence of the therapist–patient relationship? Is insight overrated in creating therapeutic change in contrast to reparative or emotionally corrective experiences? Is setting firm limits on patients' demanding behavior always more advisable than gratifying their needs? Is staff conflict an inevitable result of the borderline patient's pathology or a consequence of a faulty holding environment? Is the anger of the borderline patient intrinsic to his or her pathology or an understandable response to a therapist's insensitive comments or interventions? Is it wise to opt for an individual treatment approach only or to utilize couple and family treatment in cases where interpersonal pathology is evident?

Even before I left the Cornell faculty in 1981, my frequent lectures on borderline conditions to different staff groups in the New York area reflected my growing interest in the controversies raised by the conflict and deficit models. While originally relying on ego psychological, and object-relations formulations and treatment principles, I have increasingly experimented with self psychological techniques in my private practice, my teaching at New York University School of Social Work, and in other supervisory and consulting work. Kohut, who was originally concerned with the treatment of narcissistic pathology (1971, 1984), viewed borderline disorders as generally beyond the reach of self psychological psychoanalytic treatment. Others (Adler, 1985; Buie & Adler, 1982; Brandchaft & Stolorow, 1984a, 1984b; Stolorow & Lachmann, 1980; Tolpin, M., 1987; Tolpin, P., 1980; White & Weiner, 1986) have applied self psychological understanding and treatment principles to borderline pathology, but their work raises new questions. Does empathic understanding make some patients, for example those who are more schizoid or paranoid, worse? Are some patients so chaotic, impulse-ridden, or self-destructive that the therapist's use of a subjective, empathic approach that does not concern itself with objective reality can be equated to Nero's fiddling while Rome burned? Does correct empathy ever require that the therapist either confront or set limits on patients' potentially destructive behaviors, or point out their distorted perceptions? Do borderline patients require optimal therapeutic responsiveness or direct gratification of their needs as well as empathic understanding? Does an empathic approach help patients to feel better only so long as they remain in treatment and leave their basic pathology untouched, thus promoting prolonged therapeutic dependency? Can self psychological principles and techniques be utilized in short-term and crisis-oriented therapies? Is it possible to treat couples and families self psychologically?

In my view, no theoretical model, in itself, does justice to the complex developmental needs and problems of borderline patients, nor is it possible to present a completely integrated or unified set of guidelines for working with this population at the present time. A flexible and experimental rather than a doctrinaire approach to their treatment is necessary. I believe that it is most useful to think of borderline pathology as reflecting a range of developmental difficulties that necessitate highly individualized and attuned therapeutic interventions. It is likely that many different approaches are useful and that one may be more suited to a particular patient than another. Borderline individuals can be helped significantly to overcome the disastrous effects of their early deficits. It is the "goodness" of the fit, however, between the therapist's interventions and the patient's developmental needs that is most crucial to successful treatment.

THE FOCUS AND PLAN OF THE BOOK

This book is intended to be a resource book and guide for practitioners and trainees in all the mental health disciplines. It embodies a comparative approach to the nature, development, and treatment of borderline disorders, and while it will present some of the main current theoretical models, the book will focus on the practical application of theory to the clinical situation. Of necessity I have chosen to discuss selected perspectives in depth rather than to present the contributions of all those theorists who have written about this subject. I have tried to translate complex concepts in ways that can be readily assimilated by the range of mental health practitioners who work with the borderline population. The book also contains numerous examples illustrating the principles and techniques of different treatment approaches. The case material comes from a variety of sources and has been disguised to protect confidentiality.

The book is divided into two parts. Part I considers the historical background and main current theoretical views on the nature, development, and treatment of borderline disorders. Part II presents and critiques five conflict- and deficit-based treatment models, describes the elements of an integrative clinical perspective in the treatment of borderline disorders, and discusses hospital treatment and couple and family treatment.

The process of helping individuals with borderline disorders attain a greater sense of personal and social functioning has been both challenging and gratifying. I have had my share of anxiety, disappointment, doubt, hope, and elation. I hope that this book will enable other clinicians to try out some new ideas, to enrich their practice, and to discover the rewards of working with this "difficult" and rewarding population.

2

The Borderline Concept: An Overview

The borderline concept is a strange one. It is difficult to imagine a more confusing name for an emotional disorder. What does it mean to a troubled individual to have a disturbance that is considered to be not exactly one thing or another? The problem with the borderline designation, however, is more than semantic. Historically, it referred to a diverse group of ill-defined disturbances that did not seem to fit traditional diagnostic criteria and were more severe than the neuroses and less severe than the schizophrenias. Only more recently has the borderline diagnosis earned its place as a distinctive category, but a lack of consensus still exists about its exact nature. Stone (1987a), for example, cites five different ways of defining the borderline category, and there are others as well.

EARLY HISTORICAL DEVELOPMENTS

The confusion about the nature of borderline pathology in the early literature stemmed from three main sources: the different vantage points of clinicians, their differing theoretical orientations, and the emergence of diverse diagnostic labels.

Borderline Personality or Borderline Schizophrenia

In psychoanalytic circles within the United States a controversy developed as to whether the puzzling pathology that clinicians were observing constituted a type of severe character pathology or a less serious form of schizophrenia. Private practitioners, who treated a healthier spectrum of patients, were perplexed by those seemingly neurotic individuals who showed marked difficulties while undergoing psychoanalysis that greatly interfered with their treatment. In contrast, hospital-based clinicians were intrigued by those persons who, despite their proneness to psychotic regression, seemed to function at a higher level than was typical for most schizophrenic patients. Very few of the clinicians from either of these two broad groupings used the actual term "borderline." Instead, more than ten different diagnostic labels were generated to describe these unusual patients (Chatham, 1985; Stone, 1980).

Adolph Stern, Helene Deutsch, Melitta Schmideberg, and John Frosch were among the private practice-based psychoanalysts who saw borderline pathology as more closely resembling some type of personality disorder. Stern is credited with initiating the term "borderline." In 1938 he identified ten characteristics of office patients that were associated with either their becoming worse, or their resistance to or lack of cooperation with psychoanalytic treatment: narcissism; psychic bleeding; inordinate hypersensitivity; psychic and body rigidity; negative therapeutic reaction; feelings of inferiority; masochism; organic insecurity; projective mechanisms; and reality testing disturbances. Coining the term, "as if" personality, Helene Deutsch (1942) described individuals who tended to use depersonalization, were passive, empty, capable of only superficial relationships, and often took on the characteristics of others with whom they associated. A contemporary of Deutsch, Melitta Schmideberg (1947) described borderline pathology as a stable form of personality disorder that was characterized by instability. She enumerated nine features of borderline patients: their inability to tolerate routine and regularity; their tendency to break many of the rules of social convention; their lateness for appointments; their inability to free associate during their sessions; their poor motivation for treatment; their failure to develop meaningful insight; their chaotic lives, where something dreadful was always happening; their petty criminal acts; and their difficulty in establishing emotional contact.

Writing later, John Frosch (1960) used the term "psychotic character" to refer to patients who shared the following characteristics:

the maintenance of reality testing; infantile object relations; a capacity to quickly recover from psychotic episodes; and primitive defenses. Frosch thought that many of these patients might never become acutely psychotic, but instead would remain in the intermediate zone between neurosis and psychosis all of their lives.

Among the well-known clinicians who saw borderline pathology as a less severe or borderline form of schizophrenia were: Gregory Zilboorg (1941), who differentiated a marginally functioning group of ambulatory schizophrenic patients; Paul Federn (1947), who observed a similar type of latent schizophrenic disorder; Paul Hoch and Phillip Polatin (1949), who identified pseudoneurotic schizophrenia, characterized by multiple and severe neurotic-like traits and underlying schizophrenia; and Gustav Bychowski (1953), who described a group of patients with latent psychosis.

Robert Knight's (1953a) views were seminal among the early efforts to apply ego psychological insights to the understanding of borderline conditions. He believed that ego weakness was at the root of these disorders, which reflected a "state" between the neurotic and psychotic levels of functioning out of which patients presumably could move. Knight identified the following borderline traits: the presence of neurotic symptoms; macroscopic evidence of ego weakness as manifested by a lack of concern for their situation, the absence of precipitating stress, ego syntonic symptoms, externalization, a lack of achievement, unrealistic planning, bizarre dreams, and confusion between dreams and waking life, and microscopic evidence of ego weakness particularly in the areas of secondary process thinking and language.

Descriptive Research

While most early descriptions of borderline disorders were based on anecdotal clinical accounts, Grinker and his colleagues (1968) actually studied a large group of patients who were difficult to diagnose and thus considered to be borderline. They identified four main characteristics: (1) anger as the main or only affect; (2) defect in affectional (interpersonal) relationships; (3) absence of consistent self-identity; and (4) depression. Grinker also described four borderline subtypes: Type I, the Psychotic Border, is manifested by inappropriate, nonadaptive behavior, deficient self-identity and sense of reality, negative behavior and anger, and depression; Type II, the Core Borderline Syndrome, shows vacillating involvement with others, angry acting-out behavior, depression, and inconsistent self-identity; Type III, the Adaptive, Affectless, Defended, "As-If" Persons, display appropriate, adaptive behavior, complementary relationships, little affect or spontaneity, and defenses of withdrawal and intellectualization; Type IV, the Border with the Neuroses, is manifested by anaclitic depression, anxiety, and a resemblance to neurotic, narcissistic character.

Psychological Test Data

The early psychological test literature on borderline patients, while not extensive, has nevertheless yielded some consensus about their test patterns. The seminal work of Rapaport, Gill, and Schafer (1945–46) concluded that the borderline group resembled neurotic patients on some of the tests and schizophrenic patients on others. More specifically, their testing pattern reflected an adequate performance with no deviant reasoning on the structured WAIS, but highly elaborated, idiosyncratic associative content and peculiar reasoning on the unstructured Rorschach (Singer, 1977).

Treatment Considerations

For many years clinicians have disagreed about whether borderline patients required supportive or intensive psychoanalytic psychotherapy. Concerned about the regressive or self-destructive potential of borderline patients, many clinicians argued that the unstructured nature of psychoanalysis and its emphasis on childhood memories, dreams, and fantasies activated their pathology and made them worse. Knight (1953b) and Zetzel (1971), for example, both advocated a highly structured, consistent, supportive, and reality-oriented treatment that maximized the patient's ego strength and did not foster regression. Zetzel felt that therapy sessions should not be held more than once a week, and that the therapist should set firm limits and refrain from yielding to patients' unrealistic demands. Despite the fact that supportive psychotherapy did not attempt "to cure" borderline pathology, it became the preferred approach for many years. Some clinicians, however, such as Eissler (1953), argued for a treatment approach that attempted to modify (cure) borderline pathology and recommended a psychoanalytically oriented psychotherapy that contained certain modifications of technique (parameters).

While many clinicians believed that borderline patients who were prone to psychotic episodes or severe impulsiveness needed long term in-patient treatment, others felt that prolonged hospitalization was regressive and should be avoided. There were similar differences of opinion about the value of medication, along with or instead of psychotherapy, and about the indications for short- or long-term intervention. The absence of research on treatment fostered continued debate on these points.

As clinical interest in the diagnosis and treatment of borderline disorders has increased within the United States in the last 20 years, five main views of the nature of borderline pathology have been put forth: (1) the conflict model, in which borderline pathology is described as a type of intrapsychic defensive structure related to faulty integration of drives, affects, and object relations; (2) the deficit model, in which borderline disturbances reflect developmental failures leading to defects in the ego or the self; (3) the descriptive research model, which views borderline pathology as a syndrome reflecting characteristics based on the study of large numbers of patients; (4) the DSM-III model, which classifies borderline conditions as a specific type of personality disorder based on observable traits; and (5) the biological model, in which borderline pathology is viewed as an affective disorder. While selected developmental concepts and treatment approaches will be discussed in more detail in later chapters, what follows is a summary of these five main theoretical perspectives.

THE CONFLICT MODEL

Despite their differing emphases, Otto Kernberg and James Masterson, along with his collaborator, Donald Rinsley, substantially agree that borderline disorders reflect a type of intrapsychic defensive organization that develops in early childhood to deal with *conflict*. Treatment attempts to modify the malformed or faulty borderline structure usually through the use of confrontative and interpretive techniques, and often in conjunction with limit-setting and an external structuring of the patient's life.

Borderline Personality Organization

Kernberg (1967, 1975, 1984) sees borderline disorders as reflecting a particular type of intrapsychic structure linked to problems in the development of early object relations. He believes that in early childhood every individual acquires one of three possible types of structural organization: neurotic, borderline, or psychotic. Each type indicates the individual's level of personality development, the most advanced being the neurotic, the least advanced being the psychotic. While borderline personality organization reflects an intermediate level of development at which an individual becomes stuck, it is not a transitional or transient position. The borderline structure becomes entrenched and fixed, and affects all later personality functioning. In his view of borderline conditions as constituting a well-delineated region between the neuroses and the psychoses, Kernberg stresses the "borderland" nature of the pathology. His conception is a broad one, which comprises a variety of personality disorders according to DSM-III-R criteria (1987).

Kernberg does not view presenting problems or overt symptoms and traits as reliable indicators of borderline conditions. While a patient's general ego weakness and "presumptive" symptoms should alert the clinician to the possible presence of borderline pathology, the following intrapsychic characteristics are essential to the diagnosis of borderline personality organization: (1) identity diffusion, in which contradictory aspects of the self and others are poorly integrated; (2) primitive defensive operations centering on splitting instead of higher level defenses centering on repression; and (3) the maintenance of the capacity to test reality despite distortions caused by defenses such as extreme forms of projection and problems in the sense of reality.

The borderline defensive structure emerges developmentally to protect the child from intrapsychic conflict caused by the child's aggression. Splitting and the related defenses of denial, idealization, devaluation, omnipotent control, and projective identification ward off the individual's anxiety about the destruction of his or her good self- and object-representations by aggressive impulses. While they are warding off conflict, however, these primitive defenses weaken the ego. Identity, superego functioning, and mature object relations are not consolidated.

Kernberg's optimal approach to the treatment of borderline patients aims at modifying their pathological defensive structure and internalized object relations in order to promote identity integration, and thereby to overcome ego weakness. The therapist attempts to clarify, confront, and interpret the patient's primitive defenses and negative transference reactions, while also preventing or controlling acting-out through firm limits and external structure, such as hospitalization. In his emphasis on therapeutic neutrality, confrontation, interpretation, and limit-setting, Kernberg minimizes the experiential and corrective aspects of the therapeutic relationship.

Kernberg (1984) also describes a special type of supportive psychotherapy that can be used with those borderline patients who cannot undergo the more expressive treatment that he clearly favors. This treatment approach departs almost totally, however, from the usual conceptions of supportive psychotherapy of which he is quite critical. It relies primarily on the therapist's confronting and educating patients about the presence and impact of their pathological defenses in order to increase their adaptation to reality.

The Split Object-Relations Unit

Masterson (1972, 1976) along with Rinsley (1975) stress the rewarding and withdrawing split object-relations part units that develop to help borderline individuals deal with their abandonment depression. Drawing on Margaret Mahler's (1971) theory of separation-individuation, they argue that maternal unavailability during the rapprochement subphase is responsible for the development of defenses against the depression, rage, fear, guilt, passivity, and emptiness that are associated with autonomous efforts. Some children experience maternal withdrawal or punishment for their independent moves and rewards for dependency. In order to maintain the connection with the rewarding object and to avoid the withdrawal associated with individuation, the child erects primitive defenses that consolidate into a borderline structure. The mother's alternating good (rewarding) and bad (withdrawing) attitudes toward the child's dependent and autonomous strivings are internalized and kept split. Later life events that are associated with independence may reactivate the abandonment depression conflict and its defensive constellation.

In treating borderline patients a confrontation of pathological defenses is used initially to make them ego alien and to block the acting-out of destructive impulses. Some patients then can benefit from a more reconstructive approach that attempts to work through their abandonment depression and to modify their internalized object relations and defective ego. Unlike Kernberg, Masterson emphasizes the importance of the therapist as a real person who actively supports the patient's efforts at individuation at certain points in the treatment.

THE DEFICIT MODEL

Instead of viewing borderline disorders as reflecting a stable defensive structure that protects the individual from intrapsychic conflict, numerous clinicians believe that borderline individuals experience developmental failures that result from *deficits*. These are gaps — missing or underdeveloped elements in their personalities. Because they show severe ego, object-relations, or self deficits, treatment must build, strengthen, and consolidate the borderline patient's internal structure. Deficit-model theorists argue that most borderline patients cannot tolerate the techniques embedded in conflict-model approaches. Instead, they stress the need for a more reparative use of the therapeutic relationship. Since structure building enables the patient to attain a higher developmental level, deficit-based treatment approaches are not the same as traditional, supportive ones that leave core pathology untouched. Representative examples of deficit models will be discussed below, and others can be found elsewhere (Chessick, 1977; Giovacchini, 1979).

Separation–Individuation Subphase Inadequacy

In their view of the progressive structuralization of the ego during early development, Gertrude and Rubin Blanck (1974, 1979) see borderline disorders as representing a range of pathology that is not always clearly differentiated from the neuroses and psychoses. Drawing on the theories of Hartmann, Spitz, Jacobson, and Mahler they argue that the specific nature of an individual's ego development is determined by how he or she negotiates each of the separation–individuation subphases in early childhood. Like Mahler, they place importance on the interaction between the child's innate equipment and the degree of maternal (caretaker) attunement. The earlier the difficulties the child–caretaker dyad encounter, the more likely the child will show severe ego impairment.

The nature of treatment is determined by an assessment of both a patient's particular subphase inadequacies and the degree of structuralization of the ego. These vary considerably from one borderline patient to another. With those who are less well structured—that is, who are at the lower and middle ends of the borderline spectrum—a more supportive, ego-building approach is indicated. While interpretations that support the patient's highest level of functioning are used, so are real object experiences in which there is "measured gratification" of the patient's needs. For those who show more internal structure—that is, who are at the higher end of the borderline range—treatment can utilize more traditional techniques.

Problems in Self-Cohesion

In Heinz Kohut's (1971, 1977, 1984) self psychological view, true borderlines display a core deficiency in the formation of the self, but, as distinct from narcissistic personalities, they cover this basic deficit with a rigid defensive structure. These structures protect the individual from close relationships that might activate their underlying fragmentation. Other regression-prone individuals appear more cohesive but still are less intact than those with narcissistic personalities (Tolpin, 1980).

Severe and protracted failures in parental empathy with the selfobject needs of the child are the causes of narcissistic vulnerability and borderline pathology. The necessary transmuting internalizations that transform archaic narcissistic needs for idealization, mirroring, and twinship do not occur. The self is arrested in its development and becomes enfeebled. It lacks cohesion, and the individual develops severe narcissistic vulnerability. The concept of narcissistic rage as a disintegration product in the face of failures in empathy replaces Kernberg's emphasis on the importance of instinctual aggression in borderline disorders. Thus, the intense anger and destructive impulses that these individuals experience are secondary reactions to narcissistic assaults rather than primary expressions of aggressive drive.

Developing his theory to address the problems of narcissistic personalities, Kohut did not focus on borderline conditions, which he saw as distinctive and more severe. He became more optimistic about the treatability of borderline individuals self psychologically over the years. Because of the threat to their tenuous equilibrium, Kohut first thought that borderline individuals could not form the stable selfobject transferences (the expression of idealizing, mirroring, or twinship developmental needs in the therapeutic relationship) that are essential to self psychological treatment. He advocated supportive psychotherapy to help these patients stem further disorganization (1971, 1977). In *How Does Analysis Cure?* (1984), however, he acknowledged that the fit between a highly empathic, self-scrutinizing, and dedicated analyst and a particular patient might help to transform what appears to be a borderline condition into a treatable narcissistic disorder. Nevertheless, he continued to believe that there are some borderline and psychotic patients who may never be able to respond therapeutically because of their severe early trauma or congenital difficulties.

Self psychological treatment requires the therapist's empathic immersion in the patient's subjective experience with the goal of helping the patient to develop a greater degree of self-cohesion. Interpretation and other technical interventions focus on helping patients to understand their selfobject needs for such things as affirmation, admiration, and soothing, as well as the failures in attunement of parents and significant others in childhood. The empathic climate and experience of the therapy strengthens the patient's sense of self as much as does its content. There are differences of opinion even among self psychologists about whether therapists should restrict their interventions to empathic understanding, or whether, as White and Weiner (1986) suggest it is necessary to meet some of the patient's selfobject needs. Nevertheless, Kohut acknowledged that empathy in itself has a corrective emotional effect on patients and is an important aspect of therapeutic cure.

The Iatrogenic Myth of Borderline Structure

Building on earlier work (Stolorow & Lachmann, 1980), Stolorow along with Brandchaft (1984a, 1984b) applied self psychological principles specifically to the problem of borderline pathology and its treatment. Opposed to Kernberg's view of borderline disorders as representing a fixed, pathological defensive organization that resides within the patient alone, they argue that what appears as borderline structure is iatrogenically created—that is, it is induced by unattuned and countertherapeutic treatment techniques. Behaviors that have been labeled by others as defenses, such as splitting and projective identification, are reinterpreted as reflecting developmental arrests. They provide an "indication of needs for specific modes of relatedness to archaic selfobjects and the empathic failures of these selfobjects" (1984, p. 356). The patient's reactions arise "in an intersubjective field—a field consisting of a precarious, vulnerable self and a failing, archaic selfobject" (1984, p. 332). Thus, the more flagrant and seemingly intractable behavior of so-called borderline patients is stimulated by the failure of the patients' environment (including the therapist) to meet their selfobject needs.

Stolorow and Brandchaft argue that even those patients who suffer from "borderline" vulnerability in the self, can also be helped to develop stable selfobject transferences with the help of a sufficiently empathic and tolerant therapist, and thus can be treated successfully with a self psychological approach. Further they do not believe that there are untreatable borderline disorders but do concede that those patients who look "borderline" are more taxing on the therapist because of their greater vulnerability to disruptions in the therapeutic process and their more catastrophic, intense, and primitive reactions.

Insufficient Maternal Holding Experiences

Seeing borderline pathology as more stable than do Brandchaft and Stolorow, Adler (1985) and Buie and Adler (1982) describe the borderline's primary deficit as an inability to evoke a positive mental representation of a sustaining, holding, or soothing caretaker. Because they have not had good-enough mothering as children, they do not develop the internal resources for self-soothing that would enable them to cope with life, and what capacities do develop are easily lost under stress.

Adler and Buie disagree with Kernberg's and Masterson and Rinsley's view of the splitting defense as central in the evolution of borderline disorders. They do not think that borderlines have internalized enough experiences with good objects to make the splitting of good and bad objects possible. Instead, they argue that borderline individuals' lack of sustaining positive introjects and their resultant fears of annihilation and abandonment are more important to their pathology than is splitting. Borderline individuals lose their precarious self-cohesion in the face of disruptions in their important relationships. Prone to fragmentation and sensitive to abandonment, they become overwhelmed by a sense of aloneness. Panic and rage reactions develop. At the same time borderline patients also have a need–fear dilemma that makes them push positive experiences away because of the fear that they will be abandoned or disappointed once again.

The borderline's need–fear dilemma must be worked through sufficiently in treatment so that a stable selfobject transference can emerge. The therapy must provide a "good enough" holding environment, especially in the beginning phase and during stormy periods throughout the treatment, so that the patient will establish and maintain a positive relationship with the therapist. Eventually, the patient internalizes the therapist as a sustaining and soothing introject and develops the capacity for evocative memory. Adler and Buie utilize, but go beyond, techniques such as clarification, confrontation, interpretation, and limit-setting. They stress the importance of the therapist's actual selfobject functions and the selective gratification of the patient's needs for contact and soothing at various points in the treatment.

THE DESCRIPTIVE RESEARCH MODEL

Setting aside the issue of what causes borderline disorders, a number of clinician–researchers sought to establish whether there was an identifiable borderline *syndrome*, a cluster of characteristics that occur together with greater-than-chance frequency and that can be discriminated from those of other patient groups (Gunderson, 1984, 1987). An advantage of this approach is that it circumvents the fuzziness and inferential clinical judgment inherent in diagnosing borderline patients on the basis of intrapsychic characteristics or treatment responses. A disadvantage is that it does not link observable patient traits to developmental theory or to the clinical situation.

This effort to identify a borderline syndrome was built on findings generated from an extensive review of the borderline literature (Gunderson & Singer, 1975). This study delineated six characteristics common to most of the borderline categories: (1) the presence of intense affect, usually depressed or hostile; (2) a history of impulsive behavior; (3) a certain social adaptiveness; (4) brief psychotic experiences; (5) loose thinking in unstructured situations; and (6) relationships that vacillate between superficiality and intense dependency. In a follow-up research project on a large number of patients, in which they used the Diagnostic Interview for Borderlines (Kolb & Gunderson, 1980), Gunderson and Kolb (1978) discriminated a group of borderline patients on the basis of these traits. It is interesting to note that in a study comparing Kernberg's and Gunderson and Kolb's diagnostic methods (Kernberg et al., 1981), it appeared that while there was considerable overlap between the two approaches, Kernberg's criteria were more inclusive in that they applied to a larger spectrum of patients.

In an update of his work, Gunderson (1987) offers the following revised characteristics of the borderline syndrome: (1) low achievement despite talents and capacities; (2) impulsiveness, particularly in the areas of substance abuse and sexuality; (3) manipulative suicide attempts that seem to represent a cry for help; (4) heightened affectivity involving multiple intense and negative feelings and the absence of satisfaction; (5) mild psychotic experiences reflecting paranoid ideation, depersonalization, or brief regressions during treatment; (6) high socialization that often represents difficulty being alone; and (7) disturbed close relationships that reflect instability and intense attachments of a dependent, manipulative, masochistic, and devaluing nature. While referring to this syndrome as a personality disorder, Gunderson differentiates it from the DSM-III borderline classification discussed below, which he describes as not adequately clinically based.

While the borderline syndrome concept is not tied to a particular developmental perspective or treatment approach, Gunderson (1984, 1987) recently described borderline pathology as reflecting three possible levels of psychological functioning. This helps to explain the wide variation among diverse types of borderline patients, and why they may require somewhat different treatment approaches. He combines both a conflict and a deficit model in his understanding of borderline disorders, and his treatment approach is variable and mixed in its range of technical interventions.

THE DSM-III MODEL

After years of being excluded from the official diagnostic nomenclature, the borderline diagnosis was finally included in the *Diagnostic and Statistical Manual of Mental Disorders* (DSM-III,DSM-III-R; American Psychiatric Association, 1980, 1987), as a result of pressure from clinicians. Like the descriptive research model of the borderline, the DSM-III and DSM-III-R borderline classifications also reflect an attempt to define borderline disorders by overt signs and symptoms that cluster together without consideration of their underlying causes. Accordingly, borderline pathology is considered to be one of many types of personality disorder. In order to qualify for the borderline personality disorder diagnosis, which is an Axis II classification, a patient must have at least five of eight characteristics that include: unstable and intense interpersonal relationships; impulsiveness; affective instability; inappropriate, intense anger or lack of control of anger; recurrent suicidal threats, gestures, or behavior, or self-mutilating behavior; marked and persistent identity disturbance; chronic feelings of emptiness and boredom; and frantic efforts to avoid real or imagined abandonment.

While the DSM-III classifications represent an attempt to arrive at clear-cut, identifiable, nonoverlapping criteria for the borderline designation, many clinicians have criticized its underlying conception of borderline pathology as a single type of personality disorder, its specific criteria, its neglect of developmental grounding, and its lack of clinical utility (Gunderson, 1987; Kernberg, 1984; Kroll, 1988; and Stone, 1987a). In a study comparing diagnoses based on the DSM-III and structural (Kernbergian) models, Blumenthal, Carr, and Goldstein (1982) found that while there was considerable overlap between the two models, the DSM-III approach was narrower in its view of borderline than the structural model.

THE BIOLOGICAL MODEL

A major perspective in the early study of borderline disorders saw them as linked genetically to schizophrenia (Kety et al., 1968). The recent differentiation of borderline from schizotypal personality disorder in the DSM-III and DSM-III-R (those in this latter category more closely resembling patients who might have been described as borderline schizophrenics previously) has shifted attention away from seeing borderline personality as a variant of schizophrenia. According to Stone (1987b), however, there is a substantial amount of evidence that

supports the connection between schizotypal personality and schizophrenia.

At the same time, there has been increasing interest in studying the
relationship between borderline personality and affective disorder
(Akiskal, 1981; Klein, 1977). Many clinician–researchers argue that
borderline personality reflects an underlying mood disorder with a
biological rather than an environmental or developmental etiology, that
its appropriate treatment is therefore pharmacological, and that it will
abate if the mood disorder is treated. While it is beyond the scope of
this chapter to review this research, Kroll's (1988) recent comprehensive summary of the main findings in this area concludes that while
there is some evidence of a link between depression and borderline
personality in many cases, its nature is unclear, and the evidence for
viewing borderline pathology as a form of affective disorder is not
conclusive. Some patients may show a depressed personality that is
rooted in developmental difficulties. Others may have a more acute or
episodic mood disorder as well, and still other borderline individuals
appear not to suffer from a depressive syndrome at all, but may reflect
the impact of a traumatic upbringing, punctuated by physical and
sexual abuse.

Likewise, Kroll does not find the studies of the pharmacological
treatment of borderline disorders with anti-depressant drugs compelling, except in those instances where there is clear-cut evidence of an
affective disturbance in addition to a personality disorder. Despite
Kroll's critique, however, the complex and more than casual relationship between depression and borderline disorders warrants further
scrutiny.

Another link between biological factors and borderline disorders
lies in the area of neurocognitive impairment. Palombo (1982, 1987)
draws attention to the likely importance of such deficits in the genesis
of borderline disorders in children. This issue has been ignored largely
because the theories about borderline development have been based
primarily on adults.

THE SOCIAL CONTEXT

Individuals and families are not isolated from the social environment,
which exerts an impact on personality development, coping and
adaptation, and psychopathology. While there is no evidence to suggest
that minority group members are more prone to developing borderline
disorders, there is general agreement that societal oppression, discrim-
ination, prejudice, socioeconomic deprivation and lack of opportunity,

and absence of positive role models engender low self-esteem, self-hatred, and negative self-concepts that complicate character development and identity integration. Attuned parenting and the presence of other familial and environmental supports will cushion some, but not all, individuals from the assaults of the social environment.

Blacks and Hispanics, other ethnic and racial minorities, women, and gays and lesbians are some major examples of groups within the society who are vulnerable to identity diffusion resulting from cultural conflict, feelings of dissonance or difference, and the taking in of unfavorable societal attitudes. The achievement of a stable and integrated identity is more difficult when, at an early age, an individual does not know where he or she belongs culturally, or learns that crucial aspects of his or her experience are demeaned, derogated, and often punished by the larger society.

In discussing ethnic minority borderline clients, Comas-Diaz and Minrath (1985) comment on the strains of biculturalism that may create or reinforce split images of the self, loss of centrality, confusion, fear of dissolution, and identity diffusion. Chestang (1972) describes the sense of worthlessness, inadequacy, and impotence, that forms the experience of many blacks as a consequence of extrinsically imposed devaluation. Lewis (1984) identifies the rampant feelings of self-alienation and internalized homophobia in lesbian women that result from their externally inflicted negative labeling of their same-sex interests. Thus, it can be argued that the development of symptoms such as depression, substance abuse, and suicidal behavior may be a consequence of efforts to cope with identity conflicts that stem from conflicts between the individual and society.

Rigid and narrow role expectations are another source of potential identity difficulties. Feminism has raised our consciousness regarding the adverse impact on women of societal prescriptions for what is appropriate for them to feel, think, and achieve. Dependence and helplessness, self-destructive behavior and self-directed anger, feelings of worthlessness, and a pervasive sense of hopelessness are the direct results of societal attitudes and policies that impose constraints on women.

The impact of poverty and the lack of social justice, which deprive people of necessary resources and opportunities, engender feelings of rage and impotence. These reactions are compounded by the threat of violence, real or imagined, against all those who are different, which often leads to fear, suspiciousness, and at times retaliatory aggression.

Lastly, it is important to consider the role of traumatic events on personality development and psychopathology. Walsh (1977) and Goldstein (1981a) each note the large percentage of borderline patients who have experienced parental loss and/or other separation stresses.

Goldstein (1983) comments further on the multiple external stresses due to employment problems, financial instability or dependence, career pressures, physical or mental illness, geographic changes, and nonsupportive extended family relationships that have affected the families of borderline patients. There has also been increasing attention paid recently to the role of sexual abuse in the histories of female borderline individuals (Herman et al., 1989; Kroll, 1988; Wheeler & Walton, 1987).

CONCLUSION

The study of borderline disorders over the years has led to diverse conceptions of what they are and how they should be treated. In the absence of research on the process and outcome of different therapeutic models with borderline patients the clinician has no simple way of deciding which view is "correct," or of reconciling often contradictory treatment recommendations.

This review of the borderline concept brings important questions to the surface. Has the quest for a singular definition of and treatment approach to borderline disorders obscured the fact that there may be a range of developmental pathology between the neuroses and psychoses that requires different types of interventions? Is it better to use the borderline designation broadly to refer to all of these disturbances or to use it narrowly to encompass only some of this pathology? Should we discard the term "borderline" altogether in favor of a more individualized approach to understanding the nature of a specific patient's developmental needs and problems? More importantly, how do we deal with the nature of the impact that different explanatory frameworks have on what practitioners observe? Our theoretical beliefs and therapeutic interventions themselves may contribute to an individual's seeming pathology and to the patient's behavior in the treatment process. This fact imposes an awesome responsibility on clinicians to insure that our knowledge base serves our patients rather than perpetuates or aggravates their difficulties.

3

Major Characteristics of the Clinical Picture

How can practitioners recognize borderline patients? In their representations of the main clinical features of borderline disorders the five conceptual models (conflict, deficit, descriptive research, DSM-III, and biological, as described in Chapter 2) emphasize different, although often overlapping characteristics. They also rely on diverse sources of data on which to base a diagnosis: information about the patient's past and present functioning; transference and countertransference reactions; intrapsychic processes as revealed in the treatment situation; and overt symptoms and traits. Further, two distinctive research tools have been developed for diagnostic purposes: a semistructured interview that contains questions regarding selected areas of the patient's history and current functioning (Kolb & Gunderson, 1980), and a clinical interview that focuses on patient reactions that reflect intrapsychic structural criteria (Kernberg, 1977).

Drawing upon the various models that have been put forth, this chapter will discuss and illustrate the main features of borderline disorders as they are experienced by the patient, significant others, and in the clinical situation.

IDENTITY DISTURBANCES

A stable and integrated identity is one of the hallmarks of a relatively well-functioning personality. There is general agreement that individuals with borderline disorders show a range of characteristic identity disturbances although there is a difference of opinion about their exact nature. The DSM-III-R relies on easily observable manifestations, such as an individual's career uncertainty, gender confusion, or interpersonal problems as evidence for such difficulties. Other writers, however, look at more complex indicators. For example, Kernberg (1975, 1977) has described identity diffusion, which exists when different and often contradictory experiences and perceptions of the self are poorly integrated. His assessment of identity diffusion focuses on sometimes subtle features in the patient's self-presentation during the treatment process as described below.

1. Borderline individuals' descriptions of themselves often tend to be confusing, conflicting, vague, or unidimensional. While conveying many facts about themselves, their communications do not "add up." Opposing ideas and feelings cannot be reconciled. They tend to portray themselves either as "all good" or "all bad," so that it is difficult to get a three-dimensional sense of who they are. Some have difficulty giving meaningful information because their descriptions of their own attitudes, feelings, and experiences lack depth and feeling, or because they go from topic to topic without reflecting on the significance of what they are saying.

2. Many borderline individuals are unpredictable. They lack continuity and sameness in the ways they present or experience themselves over time. These changes do not seem to be dependent on external events. Borderlines act differently even in similar circumstances. Each self-presentation is genuine but represents only one facet of the person, who may, seemingly without reason, demonstrate abrupt and radical shifts in feelings, attitudes, and behavior within hours, days, or weeks. Borderlines tend to perceive and experience others as changing even when they are remaining constant. They do not recognize that others remain the same and it is they who change (Goldstein, 1984).

3. Possessing a highly inflated or depreciated self-concept or alternating between them, borderline individuals have difficulty acknowledging any characteristics, thoughts, or feelings that violate their particular views of themselves. While some do express confusion about their fluctuating self experiences, they ward off their inner turmoil through compulsive activity, sex, addiction, and other forms of self-destructive behavior.

4. Some borderline individuals literally take on the identities of certain others with whom they associate. They define themselves in terms of how others see them. Their interests, values, mode of dress, and mannerisms shift as the nature of their attachments change.

In the case of Amelia, a 40-year-old graduate student in the education field, identity diffusion was evidenced by her confused and somewhat fragmented discussion of her plans upon graduation. In an early therapy session she spoke at length of her resolve to move to the southwest in order to improve her chances of meeting men. Without any apparent transition she stated that she had just written for applications for advanced training in New York City and spoke enthusiastically about the prospect of refining her skills. Amelia did not seem troubled by what seemed to be her contradictory plans. In her next session she announced that she had visited a friend in a small "arty" community in Pennsylvania over the weekend and had arranged to move in with her over the summer while she looked for a place to stay permanently. She spoke of her hatred of New York City, her desire to get away, and her plan to return to her painting career, a pursuit she had left suddenly several years before after some moderate success. When the therapist commented that Amelia seemed to have many different and conflicting plans for the future, Amelia angrily said she didn't know what the therapist was talking about. "Do I have to follow the 'straight and narrow' path? What's wrong with my taking some time off and doing what I like?" When the therapist responded that she was confused by Amelia's accusation that it was the therapist who was opposed to her move to Pennsylvania since Amelia, herself, had spoken enthusiastically of relocating to Arizona or of seeking further training in New York, Amelia said that she had given up those plans and was in a different place: "Are you going to help me deal with this or what?" When Amelia came to her session the following week, she reported having had dinner with a friend of hers who was very pleased with the school that she was attending in New York. Following their meeting, Amelia had made an appointment for a personal interview there in order to learn more about her prospects for gaining admission in the fall. The bewildered therapist asked Amelia what had made her change her mind about going to Pennsylvania. Amelia answered, "I don't need a reason. This is how I am." The therapist asked if Amelia ever felt confused by going in so many directions at the same time. "Not really. I usually know what I want to do and if I change my mind, then I go after something else." When the therapist wondered aloud if Amelia ever tried to weigh the pros and cons of the various alternatives facing her, Amelia ignored her comment and changed the subject. It soon became clear that Amelia's fluctuating plans corresponded to shifting and contradictory self-representations that were not integrated. Sometimes she saw her most important goal as being married, and she was willing to abandon her professional aspirations in order to attain this end. She felt that this would earn her mother's respect. At other times she longed to realize her artistic potential and to give up the material world. She saw this course as being irresponsible but liberating. At other times Amelia saw herself as following in her deceased father's footsteps professionally in order to carry on a family tradition. Amelia's shifts also showed her tendency to adopt the views of the person closest to her at any given time. Thus, after a discussion with her mother, finding a man whom she could marry was uppermost in her thoughts. In contrast, being with friends who were professionally oriented led her to think more about pursuing further training. Spending time with her more bohemian acquaintances resulted in her wishing to follow an artistic path.

In the case of Tina, a 23-year-old secretary who lived at home with her parents and was conflicted about pursuing her sexual interests in women, identity diffusion showed itself differently. Filling the sessions with constant chatter, she hardly let the therapist get a word in unless Tina specifically requested a response. She went from topic to topic and did not convey the significance of what each subject meant to her. The therapist would try to pay close attention to what Tina was saying, but found herself getting lost in details and sudden subject changes. When she repeatedly attempted to identify or explore an underlying feeling or theme in what Tina was discussing, Tina would move on to a different topic. The therapist began to recognize several themes that reflected Tina's contradictory self-representations. She longed for her parents' approval of her lesbianism and felt unacceptable without it. At other times, however, she felt angry at her parents for being so conformist and "keeping her down." She resented being trapped by their demands on her, but felt helpless to go against their wishes, which she believed were unreasonable. In contrast to these feelings of victimization and helplessness were Tina's screaming matches with her parents that often were provoked by her defiant behavior. Tina's parents were intimidated by her, and she seemed to them anything but helpless. Likewise, Tina wanted her therapist's approval, often asking her personal questions, or for reassurance that the therapist liked her. She also made fun of, ignored, or defied the therapist when the latter attempted to explore Tina's feelings. On numerous occasions Tina's feelings of being victimized showed in her accusations of the therapist for "exploiting" her by charging her a fee and for making a living by convincing vulnerable patients they needed her.

Jeff, a 37-year-old attorney, barely made enough money to support a very meager lifestyle. Living in an apartment on the top floor of a run down, five-story, walk-up building, he envied other men who had "made it" and saw himself as a "failure" and a "fuck-up." He loved to read about power brokers whom he idealized, but had trouble containing his anger and resentment when the numerous judges who had jurisdiction over his legal cases seemed to treat him disdainfully. Longing for a close relationship, Jeff dated frequently. As soon as a woman became seriously interested in him, he found a reason to break off the relationship. Involved in the litigation of petty criminal cases during the day, Jeff loved to ride his motorcycle recklessly at night. Sometimes he would even get stopped by the police. While he wore three-piece suits at work, he always donned blue jeans and a leather jacket when he socialized, whatever the occasion. It was a long time before the therapist learned this because Jeff made it a point to dress professionally when he came for his sessions. It only surfaced when Jeff related a fight he had had with one of his girlfriends. She, by his admission, was not aware that he owned a suit, and was angry about his inappropriate attire on dates that involved her friends. Jeff was miserable in his work as a lawyer, but felt it made him seem respectable. He described how getting dressed in the morning made him feel like he was literally taking on a false identity that he could not live up to. In contrast, wearing his leisure time garb resulted in a sense of greater comfort and power, but also a feeling of being unacceptable and on the "outside." Everything about Jeff reflected his difficulties in bringing together two disparate parts of himself. On one occasion, when the therapist had to call Jeff in order to change an appointment time, she discovered that he had two different messages on his telephone answering machine. One was very businesslike, while the other was informal and used "hip" language with middle eastern music playing in the background. Typically, when the therapist tried to explore Jeff's contradictory behavior and feelings, he became silent and non-communicative or spoke of feeling like he couldn't do anything right.

While some borderline patients never "take hold" of a viable identity, as evidenced by problems with commitment in many areas of their lives, others show better functioning on the surface that hides their underlying identity disturbance. The particular nature of this difficulty may initially mask its presence. Few borderline patients announce, "I am having a problem with my identity." Likewise, they generally have difficulty giving a reliable account of themselves and others, or may reveal only one aspect of themselves at the time they enter treatment. Sometimes the confusion that clinicians experience in their early work with borderline individuals is indicative of the presence of their identity problems.

SPLITTING AND OTHER RELATED DEFENSES

Despite the fact that the DSM-III-R does not make reference to defenses in its criteria for the borderline diagnosis, conflict-model theorists, in particular, view the splitting defense as the cornerstone of borderline conditions. While others have raised objections to this view (Adler, 1985; Brandchaft & Stolorow, 1984a, 1984b; Stolorow & Lachmann, 1980), it seems important to consider how splitting and the related mechanisms of denial, projective identification, idealization, devaluation, and omnipotent control are thought to be manifested in borderline individuals.

The ability to recognize and tolerate ambivalent feelings about oneself and others is an important characteristic of adaptive functioning. It is associated with the development of self- and object-constancy, in which a person has the capacity to retain internal representations of the "good" self or the "good" object in the face of negative feelings and experiences, frustration, or in the object's absence. Those persons who have attained object constancy can become angry at loved ones without feeling that they are all "bad." Likewise, such individuals do not feel like "bad" people for having hateful feelings. In more neurotic personalities, certain impulses become associated with conflict and are defensively warded off from consciousness. For example, rather than experience anger at her husband, a wife may repress her hostility, which remains unconscious. She also may develop a reaction formation in which she becomes more solicitous toward him. Kernberg (1975, 1977) has argued that borderline individuals neither tolerate nor repress conflicted feelings and impulses. Instead, they use splitting, which involves the keeping apart of two *conscious, contradictory self- or object-images,* and other lower level or "primitive" defenses. These mechanisms protect them from the anxiety associated with the destruction of the "good" self; object-representations by the "bad" self; or object-images. Borderlines bring the tendency to utilize this defense with them to all life transactions and it is manifested in the following ways.

1. Borderline individuals cannot simultaneously experience contradictory feeling states, such as love and anger or admiration and disappointment. Thus, they tend to perceive themselves and others in extreme or unidimensional ways. Often their feelings and perceptions shift without any precipitant, or as a result of seemingly minor frustrations so that someone who is viewed as all "good" suddenly is seen as all "bad." At any given moment, however, these polar feelings do not influence one another. Thus, even if a therapist has been attuned and responsive most of the time, a lapse of sensitivity will be experienced as total. Likewise, no amount of previously experienced professional acclaim to bolster a person's self-esteem can prevent feelings of worthlessness and failure in the face of even a small career disappointment. In both instances, past performance has no reality.

2. Selected personality traits are associated with "goodness" or

"badness" and these become involved in splitting. For example, one can view assertiveness negatively and compliance favorably. Such an individual may acknowledge his or her submissiveness and coopera- tiveness while denying the existence of independent or rebellious thoughts, feelings, or behavior. These "bad" qualities are not uncon- scious, however, and generally are expressed in aspects of the individ- ual's behavior while remaining "split off" from his or her self-concept.

3. Generally unconcerned about the blatant contradictions in the ways they experience themselves, borderline individuals do not worry about or try to resolve these discrepancies. They rationalize them or become angry or defensive if these are pointed out. Thus, confronting splitting can trigger anxiety and lead to impulsive acts.

4. According to Masterson and Rinsley (1975), borderline indi- viduals show a more specific type of internal split. Their autonomous strivings, which have become associated with maternal rejection constitute a withdrawing part-object-relations unit. This is split off from a rewarding part-object-relations unit in which their dependent behavior has become connected to maternal approval. Thus, autonomous behavior brings forth fears of abandonment. Regressive yearnings relieve depression but ultimately lead to engulfment and thwart autonomy. The activation of these split units interferes with borderline individuals' personal and social functioning and may be triggered by separations, close relationships, and demands for greater autonomy.

Other common borderline defenses that are related to and rein- force splitting are: (1) denial, in which there is an inability to acknowledge selected aspects of the self or of others that conflict with one's image of the self or of others; (2) idealization, in which there is a tendency to see oneself or others as totally "good" in order to ward off more negative, frightening, and potentially destructive impulses; (3) devaluation, in which there is a penchant to see oneself or others as all "bad"; (4) omnipotent control, in which a person with a highly inflated sense of self attempts to control others totally; and (5) projective identification, in which a person continues to have an impulse, generally an angry one, which, at the same time, is projected onto another person, who then is feared as an enemy who must be controlled. Individuals who utilize this mechanism in treatment, in order to rid themselves of unacceptable hostility, still experience their own anger but feel it is a justifiable reaction to the therapist, who becomes the target of their projections. Their controlling behavior induces intense and usually angry countertransference reactions along with counteraggressive responses, submission, or withdrawal.

In the cases of Amelia, Tina, and Jeff described earlier, the presence of splitting could be inferred from the ways all three patients warded off the therapist's repeated efforts to explore their various contradictory self-presentations. Amelia tended to become angry and attacking, and justified her reactions in a rather unconcerned way as if they merely reflected her usual mode of functioning. Tina seemed either to ignore the therapist's interventions altogether or to become provocative and accusatory. In contrast, Jeff felt criticized and misunderstood, and became more depressed and withdrawn.

Splitting manifested itself differently in the case of Ron, a 25-year-old, unemployed actor. He had seen numerous male therapists for short periods over the past 8 years since dropping out of college. Each time he sought treatment he quickly developed an admiring attitude toward his new therapist and saw him as possessing special abilities. Ron generally portrayed himself as depressed and worthless, an easy pawn for others who used and betrayed him. He seemed to evoke rescue fantasies in his therapists who gave him extra time and tried to convince him of his value. At some point in each of Ron's previous treatments, however, a seemingly minor incident occurred in which he experienced his therapists as failing him and broke off treatment suddenly. For example, Ron saw one therapist driving a Toyota rather than the Mercedes, BMW, or Porsche that he fantasied the therapist owned and felt he must not be successful. On another occasion, Ron observed with disgust that a second therapist was wearing white socks under his trousers and felt contempt for his poor taste. When a third therapist inadvertently left out one of the sessions on Ron's bill, Ron decided that he was incompetent. These situations led Ron to become angry at and depreciate the therapist after he left the session. He never actually told any of them what he was feeling. Instead, he missed appointments and eventually dropped out of treatment, despite each therapist's efforts to convince him to stay. In a few instances, he left without paying for several sessions. When the therapists attempted to collect their fees, Ron became enraged at their mercenary qualities and felt that they had no right to the money since they had not helped him. One explanation of this pattern is that Ron, who presented himself as needy, admiring, and grateful for any attention that he was given, seemed to split off the aggressive, grandiose, and envious parts of himself and idealized the therapists defensively. The idealization quickly gave way to his underlying rage when the therapists did not live up to his expectations. Projecting his anger, he came to regard the formerly "all good" therapists as "all bad." He then felt quite justified in acting aggressively toward them by devaluing and not paying them. At the same time, he would leave treatment without sharing his angry feelings, thereby in some sense attempting to preserve the "good" objects from destruction.

Meredith showed a common but more subtle variety of splitting. An extremely attractive 30-year-old woman with low self-esteem, she sought out relationships with men who made her feel desirable and special, but who also at times mistreated her. She became addicted to their charm and to the good feelings she had when she was in their presence. She was always unprepared for their explosive and derogatory outbursts at her, which would make her feel worthless. After each verbally abusive encounter she would spend some time by herself only to find herself longing for contact, and so she would renew the relationship. She was not in touch emotionally with the "bad" parts of her male friends at these times and remembered only the "good" times. Meridith did not say to herself that she had to accept the lows along with the highs. Nor was she able to tell herself that despite the positive aspects of the relationships, they were too destructive to her and should be terminated. Thus, she was not able either to tolerate the men's multifaceted qualities nor to remove herself from intolerable situations. Instead, each time she sought renewed contact she expected to see the longed for "good" object and split off her perceptions of the men's "bad" qualities. While fulfilled for a brief time, her need was soon frustrated by the reappearance of the men's undesirable traits that had devastated her.

Meredith reacted as if there were two different men — the idealized one whom she desired and the real one who disappointed her. She could not bring these two polar views of them together. Likewise, she fluctuated in her self-regard in these relationships and wavered between two positions. When the men treated her well she felt worthwhile, and when they abused her she felt like a terrible person and almost accepted the blame for having been mistreated. It was she and not they who was "bad." If she could get them to love her, then she would be "good" again.

Lisa, the 38-year-old only child of needy and depressed parents, felt paralyzed in many aspects of her life. While resenting the emotional grip that her parents had over her, she felt helpless and hopeless about ever pleasing them before they died. Her parents had married in their late 30s and now were aging and becoming more dependent on her. Earlier they had always been fearful and overprotective of Lisa, while espousing hopes that she would marry and have a successful career. Every step she took toward becoming her own person, therefore, was accompanied by self-loathing, guilt, and sabotage of her own success and autonomy. When depressed she often sought the company and reassurance of her mother. Lisa dreaded being alone the rest of her life but felt convinced that she would never marry and have children. She repeatedly became involved with men who were unavailable while finding those who were interested in her "boring." She hated her job, but found it impossible to sustain any effort toward getting further training that would enable her to move into a more gratifying position. She wanted to earn more money, but could not follow through on her plans to do so. It could be argued that Lisa, by being dependent and depressed, was being a "good" girl. She was colluding with her parents' need to have her remain a child in order to give meaning to their lives. To be autonomous, successful, and happy would be "bad" and cause Lisa to feel the threat of parental loss and guilt over her abandonment of them.

In keeping apart "good" self- or object-representations from "bad" self- or object-representations, splitting, and the other lower level defenses described above, prevent patients' identity integration. This both leads to and reinforces identity diffusion. Splitting also results in rapid fluctuations of self-esteem and tumultuous interpersonal relationships, since one's feelings toward the self and others swing from one extreme to the other. In order to recognize splitting, it is important for the practitioner to see all facets of the patient, not only the ones that the patient presents at any given moment. Borderline individuals may not be able to acknowledge or integrate fully the contradictory perceptions of themselves and others even after a long period of treatment. Clinicians sometimes make the mistake of reinforcing only the "good" aspects of the patient's self-presentation or validating the patient's perceptions of others' "bad" features. Likewise, it is helpful for practitioners to be alert to what patients may not be sharing as well as to what they reveal in the treatment. It may be necessary to reach actively for information about many aspects of the patients' daily lives because of their tendency to keep important and sometimes quite troublesome issues out of their treatment sessions. When this pattern is accompanied by impulsiveness and self-destructive behavior, it may be advisable for the therapist to maintain some contact with the patient's significant others.

REALITY TESTING AND
PSYCHOTIC-LIKE FEATURES

Most individuals are able to differentiate themselves from others and can distinguish between inner and outer stimuli. They also show the ability to evaluate their behavior, thoughts, and feelings in terms of what is appropriate to social norms. While borderline individuals show difficulties that compromise their ability to perceive themselves in non-distorted ways, they retain the capacity for reality testing unless they are in the midst of a psychotic regression (Kernberg, 1975, 1977). Their issues with reality testing manifest themselves in the following ways.

1. Some borderline individuals may show psychotic-like beliefs or a loosening of ego boundaries, but can modify their false or bizarre ideas at times. For example, they may seem convinced that they are psychic and can predict the future, and cite evidence to prove this point. They often have fixed ideas that seem almost delusional, such as the belief that they are dying of an incurable illness or that they are being punished for their success. Other paranoid ideas are common, such as the seeming conviction that others can read their minds or see their true feelings. When more reality-based explanations for their perceptions are vigorously pursued or when interpretations of the underlying reasons for their distorted views are made, such individuals usually can acknowledge them and become more realistic.

2. Because of the presence of the defenses of splitting, denial, projective identification, and so on, or their lack of sufficient internal structure, borderline individuals distort reality to some degree, but their misperceptions are rarely bizarre. For example, they may be highly suspicious of friends and associates, fail to recognize important qualities in others' dealings with them, or impute malevolent motivations to those close to them. When other alternatives are presented or when their primitive defenses are interpreted, they can usually consider that they may be misperceiving the situation.

3. Showing problems in their sense of reality, as evidenced by feelings of depersonalization and derealization, borderlines may experience themselves as being outside of their bodies, looking at themselves, or may feel as if they are walking on a strange planet. At the same time, they recognize that these experiences, while frightening, are strange. Body-image distortions, such as feeling too fat even if one is thin, are frequent. These phenomena, while seeming bizarre, are compartmentalized and do not reflect more pervasive impairments in reality testing.

4. At times some borderline individuals may become acutely psychotic, making it difficult for the clinician to differentiate between borderline, schizophrenic, and manic symptoms. In borderline patients such episodes generally are transient, lasting only a few hours, days, or weeks, and usually abate with the structure of a brief hospitalization. They do not necessarily require antipsychotic medications.

5. Sometimes, when presenting an affective disorder with or without psychotic symptoms, borderline individuals may benefit from antidepressants.

The fact that borderline individuals may show psychotic-like symptoms that yield in the face of the clinician's careful exploration of these phenomena requires the practitioner to go beyond a particular patient's self- or other's report of his or her difficulties. All too frequently symptoms may be erroneously viewed as indicative of psychosis and treated with medications which, in turn, may mask the nature of the true disturbance. This problem is compounded by the reticence to take patients off of antipsychotic medications once they are receiving them, a practice which is more than questionable given our increasing knowledge of the adverse effects of many drugs.

PROBLEMS IN IMPULSE CONTROL

Borderline individuals are generally impulsive in one or more areas of their lives. Their impulsiveness may be chronic and seemingly without environmental triggers, or episodic in response to internal or external events, such as blows to self-esteem, loss, or the threat of abandonment. Often it shows itself in one of the following: alcohol and drug abuse; eating disorders; at risk sexual behavior; suicidal threats and acts that are often of a manipulative nature; financial mismanagement or gambling; other forms of self-destructive behavior; physical abuse; and violence. Borderline individuals' impulsiveness contributes substantially to the turbulent, unpredictable, and crisis-ridden nature of their lives and to management difficulties during treatment. For example, impulsive individuals who utilize splitting, and thereby come to view a friend, lover, or therapist who frustrates or disappoints them as all "bad," may break off their relationships suddenly. Other examples might include a man whose self-image requires that he be perfect, who may become so angry at his manager's criticism of him that he quits his job without concern about the impact of the loss of income; a woman whose self-esteem is dependent on her boyfriend's love, who may suddenly take an overdose of sleeping pills upon learning of his infidelity; a patient for whom a therapist's vacation may precipitate episodes of promiscuity or substance abuse; or a spouse, whose failure to gratify her husband's sexual demands may result in his becoming verbally and physically abusive.

Some borderline individuals are quite over-controlled except for severe episodic outbursts. For example, it is not uncommon for those who protect an idealized and perfectionist self-image through denial and/or splitting off of angry or other unacceptable feelings to have a sudden breakthrough of self-destructive impulses, without warning, in the face of experiences that shatter their self-concept or precarious self-cohesion.

Because borderline individuals may present only one facet of their functioning or one side of themselves initially and at certain points in the treatment, their degree of impulse control may be hard to assess. A therapist may be unaware of more negative or problematic aspects of the patients' lives. For example, a man who appeared to be making progress in treatment only revealed that he was gambling heavily and accumulating an enormous debt when he couldn't pay for the treatment. A woman who focused on her marital difficulties during each session shared the fact that she was beating her 5-year-old son only after her mother threatened to call the therapist.

The therapeutic process itself stirs up underlying impulse control difficulties. A male patient became so angry at the therapist for having rejected his sexual overtures, that he attempted to break a chair in the therapist's office. The same patient became so incensed at the therapist's refusal to answer his requests for personal information that he tracked down the therapist's home address and stationed himself outside the therapist's house over the course of a weekend. Another female patient reported that she would become so agitated by the therapist's attempts to interpret her angry feelings toward him that she would "drink myself into oblivion" after each session.

Because problems in impulse control may be so severe as to threaten on-going treatment, it is crucial for therapists to recognize patients' potential for impulsiveness early in the treatment and to help them find ways of managing their impulses. When a practitioner has some reason to suspect that impulsive and self-destructive difficulties may be a part of the clinical picture, it may be advisable to seek out information about important areas of the patient's functioning, even if such material is not spontaneously offered. In some instances it may be useful for the therapist to establish linkages with others in the patient's life during the treatment process (with the patient's knowledge) in order to be cognizant of what is occurring. Problems in impulse control that are chronic, repetitive, or that are stimulated by intensive psychotherapy itself may be life-threatening either to the borderline individual or to those around him/her. Such problems may necessitate hospitalization, residential treatment, or the use of other types of external structure. Even within a more protected environment, there are some borderline patients who present such severe management problems that they exhaust the staff or agitate and endanger the entire patient group.

PROBLEMS IN ANXIETY TOLERANCE

Borderline individuals characteristically have difficulty managing anxiety and any increase in stress may be experienced as disorganizing or overwhelming. Some borderline individuals are either anxious most of the time, or they have recurrent, disabling bouts of diffuse anxiety. For example, they experience dread when they get up in the morning, or they have sleep disturbances, in which they awake in the middle of the night. One female patient became sleepless and agitated at 3 a.m. and had to eat a small meal in order to soothe herself. Often, borderline individuals experience panic reactions intermittently in response to life events, especially in dealing with separations from the therapist and significant others. They may engage in compulsive, impulsive, or self-destructive behavior as a means of dealing with their anxiety. A woman patient became so acutely anxious upon leaving the therapist that she called her from a nearby telephone booth within minutes of the end of the session. Not knowing the therapist's whereabouts on the weekend was so intolerable for her that she could barely sleep. This same individual became so unsettled by a childhood memory that she began a cycle of binge eating and vomiting that continued for a week until she saw the therapist again. A male patient became so fearful that he might be rejected by a woman he was dating that he began to pace around his apartment. He could only relieve himself by canceling the date and going to a movie where he engaged in mutual masturbation with a strange man.

PROBLEMS IN AFFECT REGULATION

Borderline individuals have difficulties tolerating and modulating strong affects and feelings. This problem manifests itself in several ways.

1. They often show a rapid escalation of feeling states so that, for example, irritation becomes rage; sadness becomes despair; loneliness becomes aloneness; and disappointment becomes hopelessness. They become overwhelmed by too intense positive or negative feelings and thereby feel great urgency. A male patient felt so elated and overstimulated by having received an "A" on a term paper that he began to panic and found himself driving 85-miles-an-hour. He was arrested for speeding. In another case, each time a woman began to feel that she was in love with a man she was dating she would experience a type of

manic excitement and elation along with hyperactivity and agitation so that she was unable to work or to sleep.

2. Quite labile or shifting in his or her moods without apparent reason or stimulus, a borderline individual's emotional life seems to be in great upheaval or turmoil much of the time. Seemingly happy at one moment, they can be plunged into a painful depression the next. It is not easy for those close to them to understand, track, or tolerate their fluctuations.

3. Borderline individuals frequently show intense and inappropriate anger, temper tantrums, or affect storms, in which their feelings get out of control. When these displays are coupled with impulsiveness borderlines can become frightening, physically violent, or self-destructive.

4. While having difficulty tolerating unpleasant emotions, many borderline individuals inject strong feelings into their relationships and are uncomfortable when these are calm or neutral (Kroll, 1988). Their emotional intensity evokes powerful emotions in others who may feel swept up by the relationship.

Because of the borderline's difficulties with affect regulation, some theorists (Akiskal, 1981; Klein, 1977) believe that an affective disorder underlies what appears as a borderline condition and must be treated. This is a controversial issue for which there is no clear-cut evidence at the present time (Kroll, 1988).

NEGATIVE AFFECTS

Often complaining of chronic depression, many borderlines seem to have persistent feelings of anger, resentment, dissatisfaction, and envy rather than sadness. In fact, it has been observed that anger is the dominant affect for many borderline patients (Grinker et al., 1968; Gunderson & Singer, 1975). Sometimes borderline individuals have a subjective experience of inner emptiness, which leaves them feeling bereft of positive or meaningful connections to others or even to themselves (Kernberg, 1975). It is as if their inner world has been depleted. They feel dead or mechanical, estranged from others, and without the capacity to love or care about anyone or anything. Their aloneness is not the loneliness of longing but the experience of disconnectedness, hopelessness, and futility. This sense of emptiness may be transient and episodic or chronic and pervasive. Borderline individuals may attempt to relieve this painful experience through addictive behavior or other compulsive activities, such as, in some instances, self-mutilation. This seems to reassure certain borderlines that they are alive and have feelings. Sometimes borderline individuals develop a true affective disorder in addition to the chronic depression they experience.

PROBLEMS IN SELF-SOOTHING

One explanation that accounts for borderline individuals' problems in impulse control, anxiety tolerance, affect regulation, and chronic negativity is their difficulty in self-soothing. This is thought to result from their inability to evoke the image of a sustaining, holding, or soothing caretaker (Adler, 1985). Lacking the internalization of sufficient positive experiences culminating in an internal "good" object, borderline persons are at the mercy of any upsurge of uncomfortable feelings, and are often thrown back upon their negative introjects. They have no "money in the bank" to draw upon in moments of stress. They become overwhelmed by feelings of aloneness, panic, and rage and fear abandonment and annihilation. Adler argues that this core deficit is more central to the borderline's problems than splitting. It arises earlier developmentally, since splitting necessitates that the individual has the internalized positive experiences that are then kept apart from negative ones, so that the latter do not destroy the former.

According to Adler, problems in self-soothing and with the need–fear dilemma (discussed below), rather than splitting largely account for the stormy nature of both the borderline's interpersonal relationships and of the treatment process with these patients. Once they have overcome their fears of closeness enough to engage in positive relationships, they become quite dependent on others to sustain and to reassure them that they are not alone. Clinging behavior is common. Even minor separations, such as the leaving of a therapy session, can generate panic that prompts the patient to engage in desperate efforts to make contact. Requests for personal information, extra time and additional sessions, frequent telephone calls, and efforts to prolong sessions are typical in this patient group. Vacation periods may be excruciating. Feelings of being rejected or misunderstood by the therapist can result in a devastating sense of aloneness with resultant rage. Some patients immerse themselves in activities of all sorts, or engage in addictive or other types of self-destructive behavior, in order to escape from their feelings.

FEARS OF ABANDONMENT

Borderline patients commonly show fears of abandonment. In fact, the DSM-III-R substituted "frantic efforts to avoid real or imagined abandonment" for the earlier DSM-III's "intolerance of being alone" as one of its criteria for the borderline diagnosis. The abandonment fears can be explained variously in terms of: (1) the problems in self-soothing in the face of panic, rage, aloneness, and fears of annihilation that Adler discusses; (2) the fear that autonomous behavior will be accompanied by the object loss that Masterson describes; and (3) the fear that aggression will destroy the love that Kernberg emphasizes.

These abandonment fears appear in different ways.

1. Some borderline individuals will attempt to merge with others in efforts to deny or ward off their aloneness and to reassure themselves that they will never be abandoned. This may require that they be in constant proximity to or contact with those upon whom they are dependent, and to know their exact whereabouts and/or minute details of their activities. Those close to them may experience this behavior as controlling, clinging, or possessive.

2. A core problem for most borderline individuals is their need–fear dilemma that makes them ward off or withdraw from the very positive experiences with others for which they long. In fact, they may become panicked by and attempt to withdraw from or repel those who respond favorably to them. The greater the need, the greater the threat (Adler, 1985). When the need for others remains compelling, the borderline's distancing maneuvers rarely work as a protection for very long, and they approach or try to merge once again. This oscillating cycle of clinging and distancing behavior is common to many borderline individuals.

3. When they are not feeling the urgency of their loneliness, many borderline individuals manage their abandonment fears by regulating the degree of interpersonal closeness they allow so that others are neither too close nor too distant. Sometimes this is accomplished by engaging in many superficial relationships and avoiding intimacy with any one particular individual.

4. Numerous types of performance difficulties, achievements, life cycle events that involve separations or require autonomous behavior, and even therapeutic progress can stimulate abandonment fears in those borderline individuals who equate separation-individuation with object loss.

5. Separations, rejections, or disappointments may precipitate crises for borderline individuals that lead to panic, rage, or regressive reactions. Suicidal threats and acts are common, and often seem to have a manipulative quality with respect to getting the attention of or punishing the person who has left or hurt the sufferer.

6. Some borderline individuals will go to any lengths to avoid

directly acknowledging or revealing their anger or other thoughts, feelings and behaviors that they fear will lead to the destruction of the "good" object and, thus, to abandonment. At the same time, they may act out their feelings. For example, while a patient who misses sessions or who attempts to leave treatment suddenly and prematurely may be expressing anger, these behaviors may serve to protect them and others from their aggression. If they do not see or confront the person with whom they are angry, or if they do not share the "bad" parts of themselves, they preserve (through splitting) the "good" object and "good" self.

PROBLEMS IN SELF-COHESION

Self-cohesion in borderline individuals is fragile, although this is a matter of degree. While not all borderline individuals are vulnerable to psychotic decompensation under stress, some do show this propensity. Their pathological defenses, often of a schizoid or paranoid nature, protect them from disintegration experiences in which there is a break-up of the self. In these individuals there is a profound lack of self-cohesion that leaves them susceptible to transient periods of fragmentation that can be quite disturbing. In some instances these disintegration experiences lead to hospitalization.

When in equilibrium, borderline individuals can maintain their self-cohesiveness by regulating the degree of interpersonal intimacy in their relationships. They thereby avoid the loss of ego boundaries involved in their tendencies toward merger. When their needs intensify and they actively seek out others, they become more vulnerable to the merger, abandonment, and annihilation fears that threaten their self-cohesion. Some clinicians (Brandchaft & Stolorow, 1984a, 1984b) see borderline individuals' difficulties in this area as leading them to seek out archaic forms of relating to others, as reflected in the need for idealizing and mirroring selfobjects and their fragmentation and turbulent reactions when these needs are frustrated. They believe that a therapist's ability to respond sensitively to these manifestations of narcissistic vulnerability will help the borderline individual experience greater self-cohesion. Further, they argue that much of the severe pathology that so-called borderline patients manifest actually is stimulated by therapeutic unattunement rather than being a reflection of splitting and generalized ego weakness.

Adler (1985) has described how separations, rejections, and disruptions, such as unattuned therapeutic interpretations, can provoke disintegration experiences or less severe forms of loss of self-cohesion. In contrast to Brandchaft and Stolorow, however, he cautions that the borderline's need–fear dilemma will activate their anxiety, especially in gratifying relationships, and thus, will generate turbulence even in the face of, and sometimes as a result of, empathic responsiveness.

Certain aspects of the therapeutic situation may foster psychotic regression and other extreme reactions in borderline individuals who have tenuous ego boundaries and self-cohesion. These include: therapist non-directiveness; anonymity; the absence of feedback; a focus on childhood fantasies; the patient's use of the couch that makes him or her unable to see the therapist; frequent sessions that intensify the transference; and a focus on the transference. A more active, reality-oriented, face-to-face, and here-and-now approach may be necessary with these patients although Brandchaft and Stolorow (1984a, 1984b) argue that correct empathy can prevent fragmentation in most instances.

PROBLEMS IN SELF-ESTEEM REGULATION

Self-esteem regulation is a common problem in borderline individuals. While it is natural for people to experience transient reactions of disappointment, loss, anger, and defeat in response to others, to life events that are non-rewarding or frustrating, or to one's own shortcomings, individuals with good self-esteem regulation do not experience marked or prolonged shifts in their self-regard. In contrast, those with faulty self-esteem regulation are extremely dependent upon others and external approval and recognition for the maintenance of positive self-feeling. Consequently, their self-regard is highly vulnerable and may undergo radical swings as a function of the degree and nature of the feedback they receive. Sometimes it is also contingent on their ability to live up to their own perfectionist standards.

Borderline individuals lack self-regard that is realistically based. They show either highly grandiose or devalued conceptions of their abilities and talents, and tend to feel either very entitled to special treatment or unworthy. Sometimes they fluctuate between these extremes. Because of these unrealistic qualities, it is often difficult for such individuals to get the external affirmation they require, or even to engage in pursuits that could bring such rewards. For example, one man who lived on the brink of poverty and who felt that he should have had acclaim as a writer, despite his never having completed a writing project, was unable to earn a living because any pursuit other than writing was beneath him. An attractive woman who never experienced herself as good enough would find fault with any man who showed an interest in her.

Many of these individuals are very sensitive to perceived criticism, disapproval, lack of appreciation, and insensitivity. Narcissistic rage reactions at others or fits of self-loathing and self-hate may result from even seemingly minor events, such as an unsolicited or unempathic therapeutic comment. Shame and humiliation are commonly experienced emotions. In combination with borderline individuals' impulsiveness and self-destructiveness, assaults to self-esteem can result in suicide attempts, violence, and other forms of severe acting-out.

SUPEREGO DEFECTS

Borderline individuals characteristically show incomplete superego development since the superego has neither consolidated nor been integrated within the total personality structure. It does not serve reliably as an appropriate and consistent regulator of behavior. Superego pathology appears in a variety of ways.

1. Some borderline individuals show an absence of guilt and empathy in their dealings with others and are capable of ruthless and exploitative acts, features which raise the possibility of an antisocial personality. The presence of antisocial features in borderline patients usually is a poor prognostic indicator.

2. Many borderline individuals seem to manifest a "split" in their superego functioning. They may show a high degree of impulsiveness in certain areas of their functioning or at certain times in their lives, while experiencing remorse, self-contempt, and self-recriminations as a result. They find themselves unable to stop the very behavior that they hate.

3. Some borderline individuals live by a strict moral and ethical code, but episodically engage in impulsive acts that do not bother them at all despite their obvious contradictory nature.

4. Borderline individuals frequently have strict standards for their behavior and are persecuted by their superego if they do not live up to its unrelenting demands. Some negative therapeutic reactions reflect a deepseated sense of guilt that does not permit them to enjoy life.

INTENSE AND UNSTABLE
INTERPERSONAL RELATIONSHIPS

The characteristics that have been described so far in this chapter result in borderline individuals showing a pattern of intense and unstable interpersonal relationships. Intimacy is a problem since the borderline tends to merge with or distance from others, or regulates closeness so that it is not threatening. Closeness that is attained is rarely peaceful or lasting. Moodiness, possessiveness, insecurity, and highly charged interactions are common. Fights and accusations frequently occur and are usually related to feelings of being rejected or abandoned. Feelings of victimization by others are frequent (Kroll, 1988). Impulsiveness infuses the borderline individual's relationships, which often end suddenly or are characterized by frequent break-ups and reconciliations. At the same time, separations are difficult and cause anxiety and severe depression. They may lead to desperate and often seemingly manipulative and attention-getting behavior such as suicidal threats and acts or other types of acting-out.

While tumultuous interpersonal relationships are almost synonymous with borderline disorders, Kernberg (1975) suggests that other relationship patterns also exist, particularly in those persons who show more schizoid, paranoid, or narcissistic rather than infantile, character traits. This view is consistent with Kernberg's broad definition of the borderline structure, which, he believes, underlies many different personality disorders. Kohut (1971, 1977), who distinguishes between those with narcissistic and borderline disorders, views the latter as needing to protect their tenuous equilibrium by warding off relationships. Brandchaft and Stolorow (1984a, 1984b), however, observe that borderline individuals, like narcissistic personalities, also yearn for selfobject experiences in which their early stunted needs for idealization and mirroring are revived.

Nancy, age 23, showed most of the borderline characteristics that have been described in this chapter. All of her interpersonal relationships were pervaded by instability and turmoil. She lived with her parents when she sought treatment and described caring deeply about them. She was frightened that they would die and leave her alone. She sought out their company on a regular basis and would feel left out and cast aside if they so much as went away by themselves at night, on the weekend, or for longer periods. Unable to soothe her panic, she frequently called her therapist when her parents were out or away. On these occasions she would angrily accuse the therapist of being uncaring and only interested in collecting her fee. If the therapist was unavailable, or if Nancy did not get the response she seemed to need during the first telephone call, she would call again, sometimes announcing that she was canceling all of her sessions and quitting treatment. She was never able to carry out this threat because she began to feel too alone. At the sessions following these episodes Nancy would berate the therapist: "You don't give me anything. What good are you?

I don't want to need you. You should be executed for a breach of integrity. It is not fair to make money by making me dependent on you." Jealous of any attention that her older brother and younger sister received from her parents, Nancy tried to get her parents "to stop babying" her siblings. At these times she would verbally attack the parents for not appreciating her and would threaten to move out. She would engage in shouting matches with her mother, whom she felt was weak, and with her father, whom she described as irrational. In sessions she would cry and speak of her hatred of them. If the therapist empathized with her feelings Nancy would accuse her of trying to discredit her family. Sometimes when she would arrive home she would call the therapist to say that her mother had apologized to her and everything was fine. With several female lovers over a several year period she fluctuated between feelings of intense love and elation and the depths of despair about ever finding a close companion. Intimate relationships aroused jealousy, possessiveness, rejection, and fears of abandonment and reflected frequent upheavals. When involved with someone she often left telephone messages for the therapist in which she first announced that she was very happy and looking forward to seeing her new lover (Emily, for example), and then she would call again to say that Emily had been late for their date because she had had lunch with a friend and so Nancy had broken off the relationship. She wasn't going to take Emily's mistreatment of her any more. Finally, she would report that she and Emily had reconciled. It seemed as if she felt more positive toward Emily and her other lovers when they were apart during the week. She yearned for closeness at these times, but after spending time with them Nancy would become bored and distant. She then would accuse them of not loving her. There was very little calm time. She experienced all of her close relationships as tenuous, did not trust what anyone felt toward her, and marshaled evidence to justify her beliefs. For many years during her treatment she was unable to recognize how changeable she was and how she drove those close to her to distraction. This pattern was also evident in the therapeutic relationship. Nancy wanted the therapist to share her every thought and feeling. She claimed to love the therapist and spoke of her gratitude to her. These feelings were soon interrupted by Nancy's depreciation of, rage at, and efforts to be independent of the therapist. Frequently, she accused the therapist of either wanting to control her or to be rid of her. At times Nancy seemed to be convinced of the therapist's malevolent intentions and would treat her like an enemy. She became quite paranoid and her self-cohesion faltered. These occasions seemed to be precipitated by too much merging either in her relationship with the therapist or with her lovers. At work, Nancy's problems with self-esteem regulation were evident. Often she felt she was specially talented, too good for her job and the salary she was being paid, and generally unappreciated by her boss. Alternatively she felt inadequate, noncreative, and feared she would never be able to find another good job. Usually she would become more self-deprecating if she was not able to live up to her own perfectionist expectations. Despite these swings in her self-esteem, Nancy appeared to manage her work responsibilities well. Her impulsiveness was confined to her close relationships and she was not basically self-destructive. She showed no antisocial tendencies and, in fact, prided herself on her integrity, often holding very idealistic and self-sacrificing attitudes that were at odds with her self-interest.

CONCLUSION

Drawing on various conceptions of borderline disorders, this chapter has discussed and illustrated their main characteristics. These include: identity disturbances; splitting and other related defenses; reality testing and psychotic-like features; problems in impulse control, anxiety tolerance, and affect regulation; negative affects; problems in self-soothing; fears of abandonment; problems in self-cohesion; problems in self-esteem regulation; superego defects; and intense and unstable interpersonal relationships. Borderline individuals do not necessarily show all of the features discussed in this chapter. Likewise, they may vary with respect to the degree to which a particular trait may be evident. Some of these characteristics may be evaluated relatively easily on the basis of the patient's history and current functioning. Others may require more extensive exploration and observation. In many instances it may also be necessary to obtain information from those close to the patient during the assessment phase as well as at other times during the treatment process.

4

Developmental Theory of Borderline Pathology

Varying perspectives on borderline development have been put forth. Utilizing classical psychoanalytic concepts, some clinicians (Abend et al., 1983) emphasize the link between neurotic and borderline disorders. Most views on the etiology of borderline disorders, however, stress the uniqueness of borderline pathology and apply newer theoretical conceptions to explain its origins. Contributions from ego psychology, object relations theories, and self psychology, as well as from research on infants and children and their interactions with the world, have reshaped our understanding of early development and the origins of severe psychopathology.

Developmental hypotheses about the causes of borderline disorders vary in the degree they derive from what Stern (1985) calls "the clinical infant" or "observed infant" perspectives. The former is a retrospective creation, resulting from what (usually) adult patients with varying types of psychopathology recall of their early childhood experiences during the course of treatment. It is influenced by the patient's subjective experience and memory of his or her past, the nature of the patient-therapist relationship, and the therapist's point of view. The "observed infant" perspective is a more here-and-now phenomenon in which an infant's behavior is examined at the time it actually occurs. It identifies a range of early behavioral patterns that may be linked to later personality functioning and clinical disorders.

INTRODUCTION

Freudian theory derived from clinical work with adults and focused mainly on explaining their neuroses and neurotic characters. Freud thought that unresolved Oedipal conflicts centering on the expression of sexual and aggressive instincts were at the core of these disorders, which develop in individuals who have evolved a reasonably intact intrapsychic structure. Except in isolated instances, he did not discuss the more severe pathologies. Revisions and extensions of classical psychoanalytic theory have led to a better understanding of personality development generally and of the specific nature and origins of more severe disorders. Ego psychological contributions from A. Freud, Hartmann, Kris, Lowenstein, Rapaport, and others recognized the importance of the ego's autonomous or conflict-free as well as its defensive ego functions, and the role of person–environmental transactions in the process of adaptation. They drew attention to the pre-Oedipal period during which intrapsychic structure has not yet consolidated.

Different object-relations theories developed after Freud. The term "object relations" has varied meanings. In Freudian and early ego psychological parlance it referred to the child's growing libidinal investment in others and to the quality of an individual's *actual* interpersonal relationships. The writings of the British and American object-relations theorists used the term to encompass the nature of a person's *internal* images or representations of the self and the object world, the relationships among these self- and object-representations, and the impact of these internalized object relations on the development of intrapsychic structure and interpersonal relationships. Object-relations theories show how the external world is taken in psychically and shapes the development of intrapsychic structure and personality.

Members of the British group such as Klein, Fairbairn, Winnicott, Guntrip, and others focused on the development of internalized object relations in the earliest stages of life. While not initially accepted into mainstream psychoanalytic thought in the United States, which was loyal to the intellectual leadership of Anna Freud, many of their ideas have influenced our understanding of borderline development. America-based writers such as Jacobson and Mahler built an object-relations perspective more firmly into ego psychology. While self psychology has set forth a distinctive set of ideas that focus on the emergence and development of the nuclear self and on the nature of self needs and selfobject relationships, some have considered it a type of object-relations theory. After summarizing some of the main concepts of the British School, this chapter will consider the developmental frameworks of Kernberg, Mahler, Masterson and Rinsely, Blanck and Blanck, Kohut, Adler and Buie, and Stern.

BRITISH OBJECT-RELATIONS THEORIES

A number of distinctive contributions to understanding personality development came from members of the British School of Object Relations. All of the theorists who comprise this group were interested in severe psychopathology and the pre-Oedipal period of development. It is beyond the scope of this chapter to discuss this body of theory in detail, but it will summarize the views of the major representatives of this group as they shed light on the origins of borderline pathology.

Melanie Klein

Melanie Klein (Kernberg, 1985; Klein, 1957; Segal, 1964) was one of the first theorists to focus on the pre-Oedipal period in the genesis of severe psychopathology. A child analyst, she was extremely interested in mother–child relationships. While initially placing Freud's psycho-sexual stages much earlier than he believed, she later departed radically from Freudian theory. When she moved to London in 1926 she developed her own view of developmental stages and processes, the nature of defense, and the determinants of psychopathology.

Arguing that infants possess an inborn awareness of the mother and that their fantasies always reflect feelings about and impulses toward others, Klein emphasized the role of instinctual aggression and unconscious fantasy in determining the nature of the child's perceptions and experience of early objects. Thus, it is not the real but the phantasied objects in the infant's life that determine the nature of their internal world, although the real objects may reinforce or challenge the infant's perceptions.

From birth, infants must deal with the conflict between their life and death instincts and love and hate. Envy and greed are dominant. Destructive fantasies about and impulses toward others make the infant anxious, and it fears the objects upon which it vents its anger. Rage is projected and results in persecutory fears that are heightened during the paranoid–schizoid position present in the first 6 months of life. This stage is also characterized by the use of early defense mechanisms such as splitting, projective identification, introjection, idealization, and denial that help the infant to rid himself or herself of this anxiety. In the last half of the first year of life the infant enters the depressive position in which the life instincts and love temper the aggressive drive and hate. Splitting decreases and the infant is capable of experiencing external objects as both good and bad. In order to preserve "good" objects, infants make reparation for their aggressive fantasies and impulses. They are capable of experiencing gratitude and guilt as well as mourning reactions and manic defenses. Both the paranoid–schizoid and depressive positions shape later personality development and psychopathology. They are always active in different degrees.

Fairbairn

Fairbairn (1952, 1954), who lived and worked in Scotland, rejected both Freud's and Klein's instinctually-based theories. He regarded infants as object-seeking rather than as pleasure-seeking. In a sense, Fairbairn saw the infant as born with a drive for attachment to others. He argued that personality develops as a result of interactions with real rather than fantasied objects. In addition to his stress on mothering and interpersonal relationships, Fairbairn's theory focused on the internalization of "bad" objects and the development of ego splitting. He believed that the frustration caused by failures of the external environment result in aggression that is not innate. The child's main frustrations are not feeling loved or lovable, or that its love is not welcome and valued. The inability of external objects to provide these necessary experiences lead the infant to build up a world of internal objects.

According to Fairbairn (1952, pp. 162–179), the child internalizes a "bad" object that is split into three parts. The split ego is also composed of three aspects. The parts of the object are as follows: (1) an idealized object, which is satisfying and which represses the frustrating object; (2) a rejecting object, which represents the mother's denial of the infant's needy self; and (3) an exciting object, which stimulates but frustrates the infant. The parts of the ego include a central ego, which adapts to the external world and relates to the parent as an idealized object; an antilibidinal ego, which directs aggression toward the ego and relates to the parent as a rejecting object; and a libidinal ego, which seeks out the exciting object and represses feelings of need and longing. The internalization of bad objects and the split in the ego that result from frustration become closed systems that influence further personality development and psychopathology. They prevent the individual from progressing from infantile dependence to mature dependence, and from establishing loving and satisfying bonds with others.

Winnicott

A pediatrician, Winnicott (1960) stressed the importance of "good enough mothering" and the provision of a "maternal holding environment" in the development of the healthy personality. In his view, when such an environment is lacking because of deprivation or too much "impingement" by the mother, the infant's "true" self, which represents an individual's core potentialities, becomes split off from the "false" self, which is a facade aimed at pleasing others. As the false self rigidifies, the person becomes alienated from his or her true self. Thus, the false self is a defensive organization that both "hides" and "protects" the true self at the expense of its full expression. It can be more or less severe depending on the nature of early mother–child interactions and in some instances can lead to psychosis.

In contrast to Fairbairn, who stressed the internalization of "bad" objects, Winnicott vividly described the child's acquisition of positive internalizations based on attuned mothering, as well as the ego defects that result from maternal failures. He emphasized the child's acquisition of the capacity to be alone, which he attributed to the child's experiences in being alone in the presence of an attuned other (1958). Winnicott (1953) also drew attention to the significance of transitional objects in helping children bridge their view of their own omnipotence with their realization that mother is separate and, hence, not controllable. Objects that become transitional objects are both separate from yet represent the mother, but can be manipulated by the child, thereby continuing the illusion that mother is still under the child's control.

Guntrip

Guntrip (1961, 1969, 1973), who was interested in theology, totally rejected Freudian theory on moral grounds, believing that Freud did not appreciate the more holistic and humanistic nature of man. He, like Fairbairn and Winnicott, emphasized the importance of early mothering. He argued that frustrations caused by external objects, primarily the mother, lead the infant or child to turn away from objects rather than to maintain relations with them internally. This pathology is central to the schizoid problem, which is at the heart of all psychopathology. It is characterized by: ego-splitting; a withdrawal from interpersonal relationships; attitudes of omnipotence, isolation, and detachment; hopelessness; and a preoccupation with inner reality. Not all individuals who suffer from an underlying schizoid problem function at the same level. Some have built up a neurosis that covers their basic sense of emptiness. At the most extreme end of the continuum is the person who has become completely alienated from himself or herself and who has no capacity to love, to feel understanding, warmth, or personal concern for others. Deeply hidden in such a person is his or her needy self, which is cut off from communication with the outside world.

KERNBERG'S THEORY OF OBJECT RELATIONS

Obtaining his formal education and psychoanalytic training in Chile, after his family had emigrated from Vienna when he was a child, Kernberg was greatly influenced by Kleinian theory and later, by the writings of Edith Jacobson and Margaret Mahler. After coming to the United States he wrote extensively and tried to integrate many Kleinian concepts into American ego psychology and object-relations theory, particularly as they contributed to the understanding and treatment of borderline and narcissistic pathology. His writings derived solely from his clinical work with adults. Despite Kernberg's disagreement with some aspects of Klein's thinking, he shares her emphasis on instinctual aggression, unconscious fantasy, and primitive defenses. Likewise, he minimizes the impact of the real people and events in the child's life in favor of a focus on how the child's inborn dispositions and instincts organize the nature of his or her internalization of the external world. He argues that what the child takes in psychically usually differs from the actual objects in the environment, since drives, affects, wishes, fantasies, and defenses shape and distort the child's perceptions and experiences.

Developmental Concepts

Kernberg (1976) traces the development of an individual's *internalized* object relations through a series of sequential stages that lead to the progressive structuring of the psychic apparatus and to the consolidation of ego identity. A vital and complex concept, internalization takes on different forms. Introjection is the earliest type of internalization in which the individual takes in the least organized self- and object-images under the impact of highly charged and primitive affects (feelings). Experiences begin to cluster into "good me" and "bad me" ego states depending on whether the infant is experiencing pleasurable or frustrating interactions with the environment. The resultant images, also referred to as representations, introjects, or internal objects, reflect these positive or negative ego states that are initially experienced in all consuming and sometimes frightening ways. For example, the infant may retain an ominous and powerful image of its mother's angry face that becomes associated with the infant's intense hunger.

Identification, a later form of internalization, rests on the child's ability to perceive his or her separateness from others, and the different roles each participant plays in important transactions. The little girl whose mother sings to her in a loving and soothing way when she is going to sleep takes in a positive image of the mother in relation to the child's fatigue and bedtime routines. This later shows in the pleasure she experiences when singing to her doll when she imagines the doll is tired. These early introjects and identifications may remain particularly vivid and powerful in their positive and negative impacts on later behavior and attitudes toward the self and others. Ego identity, the highest level of internalization, involves the consolidation of all of the individual's introjects and identifications into a coherent whole.

Kernberg delineates five successive stages in the internalization of object relations.

Stage 1: Normal "Autism" or Primary Undifferentiated Stage. In the first month of life the infant exists in a state of being objectless, unrelated, or undifferentiated with respect to the mother or main caretaker, although optimally the infant starts to build up a core of pleasurable experiences.

Stage 2: Normal "Symbiosis" or Stage of the Primary, Undifferentiated Self-Object Representations. During the second month of life and continuing to between 6 and 8 months of age, the infant begins to acquire a "good" internal self-object (infant–mother) image, which becomes the nucleus of the ego as a result of the mother's gratification of the infant's physical needs. The infant also builds up a "bad" inner self-object image under the impact of frustrating or painful encounters. The hyphenated term "self-object" in an object relations context connotes that the infant's internal representations of self and mother are fused or undifferentiated. This differs from the unhyphenated term "selfobject" in self psychological theory, which refers to an attuned caretaker who performs vital functions for the child that it cannot carry out itself.

During this second stage, pleasurable experiences facilitate ego development while excessive frustration generates intense anxiety. The infant tries to expel or project rather than take in or introject the resultant "bad" self-object images. While the infant begins to be able to differentiate from the mother, this capacity is quite rudimentary and tenuous.

Stage 3: Differentiation of Self- from Object-Representations. In Stage 3, which extends from the ages of approximately 6 or 8 months to 18 to 36 months, the child becomes reliably able to differentiate between self-representations and object-representations. Not yet able to experience either the self or objects in their totality, the infant cannot remember good feelings when frustrated nor bad feelings when gratified. Libidinally invested "good" self-images which now are differentiated from libidinally charged, "good" object-images, build up separately from aggressively tinged "bad" self-images that now are differentiated from aggressively infiltrated "bad" object-images. The continuing separation of self- and object-representations into "good" and "bad" reflects the child's lack of integrative capacity and cognitive immaturity at this time. Moreover, Kernberg argues that the child, who fears that his or her "bad" self- and object-representations will destroy the "good" self- and object-images, begins to experience severe conflict. Splitting and other primitive defenses (denial, devaluation, idealization, projective identification, and omnipotent control) come into play in order to ward off conflict and anxiety by maintaining the separation between "good" and "bad" self- and object-representations.

Stage 4: Integration of Self-Representations and Object-Representations and Development of Higher Level Intrapsychic Object-Relations-Derived Structures. Stage 4, which extends from approximately 3 to 5 years of age, is characterized by the child's ability to integrate both his or her "good" and "bad" self-images into a coherent self system and his or her "good" and "bad" object-images into a total and three-dimensional conception of others. The child is able to experience bad feelings toward the self or the object without losing all the good feelings. Splitting and other related defenses gradually give way to repression as the child's major defensive operation. Thus, anxiety and guilt arousing feelings or experiences become part of the unconscious rather than being split off or projected.

The intrapsychic apparatus begins to consolidate during this stage, particularly as the superego becomes more structured. Superego development involves the transformation or "toning down" of both the extremely negative self-object representations and the highly positive or primitively idealized self-object representations. The resultant internalization of more realistic self-object images within the superego lessen its harsh control over the child, substituting more appropriate demands and prohibitions.

Stage 5: Consolidation of Superego and Ego Integration. In Stage 5, which occurs approximately between 5 to 7 years of age, superego integration is completed and ego identity is consolidated under the impact of real experiences with others. A harmonious inner world, which has been shaped by interactions with external objects, stabilizes the personality and effects all later interpersonal relationships. In turn, the outside environment reinforces one's ego identity or self-concept.

The Origins of Borderline Pathology

Kernberg links the three possible types of personality organizations or structures (psychotic, borderline, or neurotic) that may develop to particular outcomes of each of the stages of internalized object relations described above. A psychotic structure (the most fragmented) arises when an individual becomes fixated in Stages 1 or 2. A neurotic structure (the most consolidated) results from successful completion of all the stages.

Stage 3 is crucial to the pathological formation of the borderline structure. Kernberg argues that the excess aggression that some children experience at this time heightens their fear of destroying "good" self- and object-representations. When such intense conflict results, they must use the splitting defense to ward off their anxiety. Unable to overcome splitting as a major defensive operation, intrapsychic structure and ego identity do not consolidate. Instead the child becomes fixated and develops borderline personality organization.

In discussing the origins of the over-abundant aggression that is central in this conflict model of borderline development, Kernberg emphasizes constitutionally-based predispositions that color the ways that children experience their caretakers, rather than the impact of parental failures and actual parent–child interactions per se. He does concede, however, that very early frustration may play a role in generating this excess aggression. Likewise, borrowing a term from Winnicott, he acknowledges that the mother who provides a good enough "holding environment" may enable the child to learn that aggressive urges and behavior will not destroy him or her, thus helping the child to overcome splitting.

The three structural characteristics that are the hallmark of Kernberg's conception of borderline personality organization originate at this time. The child who becomes fixated in Stage 3 has been able to differentiate himself or herself from others to some extent. This movement allows the child to get beyond the psychotic structure and allows for the development of reality testing and reasonably firm ego boundaries. In some instances, however, this differentiation is still tenuous and renders the person vulnerable to brief psychotic regressions under stress. Splitting and other primitive defenses continue beyond their phase-appropriate emergence and the child never acquires a realistic, three-dimensional conception of others or an integrated sense of self. Instead, identity remains diffuse and other ego functions are adversely affected, such as the capacity to neutralize anger, impulse control, anxiety tolerance, and sublimatory capacity. Thus, generalized ego weakness occurs. The resolution of the Oedipal phase is compromised and the superego remains unintegrated into the rest of the intrapsychic structure. This may reflect alternately extremely harsh and exacting or overly permissive internal attitudes. These structural abnormalities become a stable part of the personality and affect the individual's ways of experiencing himself or herself and of perceiving and relating to others.

MAHLER'S SEPARATION-INDIVIDUATION
THEORY

A psychoanalytic ego psychologist who's views evolved in harmony with those of Edith Jacobson, Margaret Mahler based her theory of personality development on naturalistic studies of child–mother interactions as well as her clinical work (Mahler, 1968; Mahler, Pine, & Bergman, 1975). She systematically shows how internalized object relations and intrapsychic structure evolve as a consequence of the child's dual efforts at *separation–individuation*. The process of separation involves the infant's gradual emergence from a fused state with the primary love object and individuation permits the development of the child's own unique characteristics.

Mahler influenced Kernberg and their stage theories overlap to a large extent. Mahler, unlike Kernberg, was opposed to Klein's minimization of the external world and underscored the crucial role of the mother's availability and attunement to the child in determining the outcome of all phases of development. Consequently, her writings have a much different flavor than do Kernberg's with respect to the significance given to the *actual* interpersonal transactions between mother and child, an emphasis more characteristic of the work of Fairbairn, Winnicott, and Guntrip.

Developmental Concepts

Mahler describes a chronologically ordered series of five developmental stages, each of which results in major intrapsychic achievements. The first two of these stages lay the foundation for the actual separation-individuation process.

Stage 1: The Autistic Phase

Until approximately one month of age, the infant lives in its own world and only fleetingly responds to external stimuli. The autistic phase can be described as a preattachment period, although the mother's attentive and attuned ministrations are necessary for attachment to occur.

Stage 2: The Symbiotic Phase

Gradually the protective shell around the infant gives way and it begins to perceive the mother as a "need-satisfying object," although the mother is not yet experienced as separate from the infant. This phase of psychic oneness extends from about 1 to 4 or 5 months of age and marks the beginning of the infant's ability to invest in and attach to another person. During this period the mother mediates between the infant and the external world, and the sensations the child experiences in relation to the mother form the core of the infant's sense of self. The mother affects the child through her sensitive and loving handling of the infant's body, her attunement to the infant's needs for physical nurture and comfort, her ability to provide soothing when the infant is in distress, and her ability to regulate and organize experience and stimuli.

The precursors of both separation and individuation occur during the symbiotic phase as the mother begins to respond to or "mirror" the infant's individual characteristics, and as the infant comes to recognize and get a "feel" for the mother who is satisfying its needs. Optimal responsiveness during this period not only helps the child to acquire a positive core self experience but also fosters separation from the symbiotic orbit.

Stage 3: The Differentiation Subphase

This stage initiates the beginning of the separation–individuation process proper. If the mother provides an adequate holding environment in the autistic and symbiotic stages, the child begins to differentiate more clearly from the mother between approximately 5 to 10 months of age. Infants are "hatched" so to speak. They look more alert, show greater interest in the outside world, become more goal-directed, and engage in more exploratory and experimental behavior. This initial differentiation is tenuous and can be easily lost if events around the child are traumatic.

Transitional objects — that is, objects that substitute for the mother through their actual association with her (by smell and touch, for example) — become important during this period. Likewise, infants often take on the mother's characteristic behavior such as stroking themselves. At about 7 or 8 months the infant seems to compare the mother visually with unfamiliar objects in what has been called a "checking back pattern," and acquires the ability to discriminate particular maternal characteristics. According to Mahler, stranger anxiety, in which infants show distress when in the presence of someone other than the mother even if the mother is also there, occurs here. This phenomenon appears to be a highly individual matter and sometimes occurs only minimally. If maternal attunement has been optimal in the symbiotic phase, the infant's differentiation subphase is more likely to be characterized by an eager curiosity rather than by fear.

Mahler did not specifically study the role of the father in the infant's development, although she regarded it as a special one, neither fully outside nor a part of the symbiotic orbit. She did believe that the father's responses to the child do contribute to the child's self- and object-representations. Abelin (1971) suggests, however, that the father's major function during the separation–individuation process is to represent the outer world and attract the child away from the pull of symbiosis. In this rather limited view the father comes to be equated with difference, excitement, and novelty and "rescues" the child from the confines of his or her relationship with the mother.

Stage 4: The Practicing Subphase

During the practicing subphase, from about 10 to 16 months of age, the separation of the child's self- and object-representations consolidates and individuation accelerates. As children become more mobile they are able to move away from the mother physically and to expand their world, optimally in close proximity to the maternal figure who is there to provide continuing support and encouragement. Although many children may show increasing efforts at individuation even when they do not experience the mother's ongoing interest and availability, their resultant internalizations nevertheless will be affected. For example, individuation may become associated with object loss.

In the early practicing subphase the child simultaneously experiences the pull of the outside world and closeness with the mother. Separation anxiety may increase until the child becomes reassured that the mother is still there. One can observe the child's initial repeated efforts to keep track of the mother even when crawling away from her, and the child's attempt to relocate the mother if she has been lost momentarily. Gradually children become more able to be on their own without seeing the mother.

During the second part of the practicing subphase children enthusiastically and even joyfully explore the world around them and may appear oblivious to the mother's temporary absence. The child's sense of power and grandiosity is at its peak. Pleasure in their rapidly developing ego functions seems to enable children to sustain transient separations from the mother that stem from their increasing efforts at individuation. The threat of object loss is present, however, and the child needs a good deal of reassurance that mother still cares. Her continuing ability to support the child's individuation while maintaining her loving availability is a vital factor in a favorable outcome to this process.

As in Kernberg's Stage 3, "good" and "bad" self- and object-representations remain separated during this period. The child experiences the mother and himself or herself as all "good" or all "bad" and is not able to retain a "good" internal representation of the mother if she is absent for long periods or otherwise frustrating the child.

Stage 4: The Rapprochement Subphase

With the maturation of the child's motor and cognitive functions and his or her increased individuation and autonomy from about 16 to 24 months of age, the child paradoxically experiences more separation anxiety. This may stem from the increasing insecurity children experience when they begin to recognize that they are not all powerful and the center of the universe. The child turns to the mother for help but fears being re-engulfed by her, makes increasing demands on the mother's time, wants to share everything with her, and craves the constant reassurance of her love while, at times, pushing her away and showing great irritability toward her. Children come to realize that their mothers are not omnipotent and that they must stand on their own two feet. At the same time the child is frightened that now he or she will be completely alone and will lose the mother's love. Mahler used the term "ambitendency" in describing this push–pull of the urgent and competing needs for closeness and autonomy that characterizes the rapprochement period.

It is difficult for many mothers to deal with this stage as their children often exhibit contradictory mood and behavioral swings ranging from a great deal of clinging and controlling to rejecting behavior. The mother's ability to accept the child's needs and even aggressive and provocative behavior while remaining encouraging and available is critical to the successful resolution of this stage (Edward, 1976). The mother must be a reliable figure on whom the child can count and with whom he or she can check out new achievements. Under optimal conditions children continue to pursue their autonomy with a greater sense of security and well-being. They gradually accept that the mother is a person in her own right with needs of her own. The child overcomes splitting and thereby internalizes and consolidates a three-dimensional view of the mother who loves and hates, rewards and punishes, and has unique characteristics. This achievement also enables the child to develop an integrated and holistic view of his or her own previously separated "good" and "bad" characteristics.

Stage 5: On the Road to Object Constancy

From about 24 to 36 months of age (and even much later) the child seems able to be on his or her own to a greater degree than previously without undue concern about the mother's whereabouts. The child increasingly acquires a solid internal representation of the mother that permits the child to pursue the full expression of his or her individuality and to function independently without fearing separation or abandonment. At the same time the child is able to experience closeness without fearing engulfment. The final achievement of object constancy implies the capacity to maintain a positive mental representation of the mother in her absence or in the face of frustration.

While Mahler focuses on infant and early childhood development, Blos (1975) suggests a second separation–individuation phase in which adolescents disengage themselves from the more infantile aspects of their self- and object-representations and acquire a more realistically based sense of themselves and their parents. This disengagement process also results in the overthrow of an archaic and rigid superego that is based on earlier idealizations of the parents, and requires that the adolescent find new love objects outside the family orbit.

The Origins of Borderline Pathology

The most pivotal concept in Mahler's theory with respect to borderline development is object constancy, which can fail to develop in the rapprochement subphase (Stage 4) due to the mother's emotional unavailability and/or lack of attunement to the child's phase-appropriate needs for separation–individuation. Instead of encouraging and supporting the child's autonomous strivings during this period, the mother emotionally withdraws from, shows negative attitudes toward, or overtly rejects the child. While having achieved some differentiation from the mother, the child has not yet internalized a stable and integrated representation of her. The mother–child dyad's failure to master the rapprochement crisis impairs the child's attainment of both object constancy and an integrated sense of self. The child becomes preoccupied with fears of engulfment and abandonment, shows difficulty modulating angry impulses, and generally shows impaired ego and superego functioning.

MASTERSON AND RINSLEY'S SPLIT OBJECT RELATIONS UNIT

Masterson (1972, 1976) and Masterson and Rinsley (1975) build on Mahler's description of the rapprochement subphase to account for the origins of borderline disorders. They also draw on Kernberg's view of the nature of internalized object relations and Fairbairn's description of a split internalized bad object. In their view, the so-called borderline mother, while enjoying her child's symbiotic phase, cannot tolerate her child's increasing individuation in the rapprochement period. She discourages the child's autonomous strivings through her emotional withdrawal or actual disapproval, while she rewards the child for his or her regressive or clinging behavior. Experiencing a terrible conflict that has two equally bad alternatives, the child may individuate at the price of experiencing depression and abandonment or remain dependent and regressed while feeling good (rewarded).

The child who becomes borderline internalizes what is termed "a split object-relations unit" composed of an aggressively charged "withdrawing part-unit" and a libidinally charged "rewarding part-unit." The "withdrawing part-unit" is composed of an attacking, critical, hostile, angry, withdrawing maternal part-object in the face of the child's efforts at individuation in relation to an inadequate, bad, helpless, guilty, ugly, and empty part-self. In contrast, the "rewarding part-unit" reflects an approving and supporting maternal part-object in the face of the child's regressive and clinging behavior in relation to a good, passive, and compliant part-self. This "split object-relations unit" affects the borderline individual's self perceptions and views of others.

The borderline ego is also split. The child escapes from the abandonment depression that would result from successful individuation through the utilization of primitive defenses and the maintenance of a pleasure-seeking or pathological ego. The reality ego does not fully develop. The child denies the reality of separation, and maintains a wish for and engages in efforts at reunion with the mother. Regressive and clinging behavior feels good because it defends against the bad feelings that would ensue if the individual were to act more autonomously. In fact, if the child (or adult) does experience actual separation or acts of individuation at various points in life, the "withdrawing part-unit" along with abandonment depression, is activated. This development, in turn, activates the "rewarding part- unit," along with more dependent behavior. It is consistent with Mahler's ideas to view earlier subphase experiences as influencing both the rapprochement crisis and its successful resolution. For example, unmet symbiotic needs can exacerbate the child's need for closeness with the mother and compromise separation–individuation. Some children may ward off their intense symbiotic wishes at the expense of closeness with the mother. Problems in differentiation may intensify separation anxiety, equating individuation with object loss. Practicing failures may lead to severe narcissistic injury when the child confronts his or her lack of omnipotence (Edward, Ruskin, & Turrini, 1981).

THE BLANCKS'S SEPARATION-INDIVIDUATION SUBPHASE INADEQUACIES

While emphasizing the decisive role that the rapprochement subphase plays in personality formation, Gertrude and Rubin Blanck (1974, 1979) draw attention to the distinctive contribution that each of Mahler's separation–individuation subphases make to borderline pathology. Thus, problems in caretaker–child interaction in the symbiotic, differentiation, practicing, rapprochement, and on the way to object constancy subphases may result in deficiencies in the ego's structuralization. Consequently, in contrast to both Kernberg and Masterson and Rinsley, the Blancks argue that there is a range of borderline pathology and that the nature of particular subphase inadequacies determine how each type is manifested. Early subphase inadequacies give rise to less structuralization of the ego and to a lower level type of borderline pathology than do later subphase inadequacies. If, for example, the child does not resolve the symbiotic or differentiation subphases fully, the borderline pathology that results may reflect longings for symbiotic union with others, fears of merger, a tendency to psychotic regression, and tenuous ego boundaries. Difficulties in the practicing period may leave the child feeling joyless in the face of autonomy or unable to individuate. If the child first encounters problems in the rapprochement subphase, the child may show more splitting along with some higher level defenses and more neurotic-like difficulties.

Among the common difficulties that the lower and middle level borderline patients show are: symbiotic longings; fear of merger; problems in self and object differentiation; faulty internalizations; insufficient neutralization of aggression; lack of object constancy; poor affect differentiation; absence of signal anxiety; incapacity for self-soothing; tendencies toward action rather than verbalization; lack of pleasure in or insufficient individuation; primitive defenses; and reliance on dyadic interactions.

The origins and range of borderline pathology accounts for the many variations one sees in the ego functioning of borderline individuals. The use of the term "subphase inadequacy" instead of the earlier term "subphase deficit" (G. Blanck and R. Blanck, 1979) connotes the idea that the negotiation of the separation process is co-determined by both mother and infant. The Blancks (1977) also make an important distinction between drive and affect that has significant implications for distinguishing between the traditional concept of resistance and what may be more adaptive efforts at preserving identity in an insufficiently structured individual. Thus, while the aggressive drive is present and may be accompanied by oppositionalism, this affect may represent the individual's effort to maintain his or her autonomy. Following this line of thought, many behaviors in which the borderline patient engages may need to be understood as reflecting their best efforts at adaptation.

KOHUT'S SELF PSYCHOLOGICAL THEORY

Originally identified with classical Freudian psychoanalysis and ego psychology, Heinz Kohut gradually evolved a distinctive theoretical model that constituted a radical departure from traditional psychoanalysis. His efforts to apply psychodynamic theory to the development and treatment of narcissistic disorders led him to reformulate many principles of development and the nature of psychopathology. Kohut's views are based on his treatment of adults, although observational studies of infants and young children are lending support to the main thrust of his ideas (Lichtenberg, 1987; Stern, 1985).

Relegating the drives and the structural model of the mind (id, ego, and superego) to the background, Kohut's writings (1971, 1977, 1984) emphasize the development of the self, which is the central organizing and motivating force in the personality. Describing a separate developmental line for the evolution and maintenance of healthy narcissism, Kohut sees the self emerging as a result of the interplay between the infant's innate potentialities and the selective responsiveness of the caretaker environment. Like Fairbairn, Winnicott, and Guntrip of the British School of Object Relations, Kohut stresses the role of actual parental empathic failures with respect to the child's emerging needs in producing deficiencies in the structuring of the self and hence, self disorders. Unlike Kernberg and Mahler, he does not subscribe to a sequential stage theory of personality formation.

Developmental Concepts

The following key concepts are important in understanding self psychology.

Selfobject

The earliest selfobjects are those attuned caretakers who perform vital functions for the newborn infant that it cannot carry out itself—for example, soothing. The infant enters the world preadapted to cue and respond to a potential selfobject milieu, and experiences its first selfobjects in terms of its phase-appropriate developmental needs without regard for them as truly separate entities.

Kohut clearly identified three main types of selfobject needs in the child's early environment: the need for mirroring that confirms the child's sense of vigor, greatness, and perfection; the need for an idealization of others whose strength and calmness soothe the child; and the need for a twin or alter-ego who provides the child with a sense of humanness, likeness to, and partnership with others (Elson, 1986). To these selfobject needs Wolf (1988) adds: the need for merger experiences with someone who is totally subject to the child's initiative and who functions as an extension of the self; the need for an adversary who provides a supportive but oppositional relationship in the service of autonomy; and the need for efficacy in having an impact on others and in being able to evoke desired responses. While not all of these selfobject needs may be gratified in a particular child's life, rewarding experiences with at least one type of selfobject give the child a chance to develop a cohesive self.

Although early selfobjects are crucial to the development of the infant's self, the need for others to provide support and sustenance continues all through life. Thus, according to Kohut, the ability to seek out gratifying selfobject experiences, in contrast to the capacity for total autonomy, is the hallmark of health (Elson, 1986). Optimally, however, the individual undergoes a transformation whereby he or she relates to others in terms of more mature rather than archaic selfobject needs.

Transmuting Internalization

The self becomes structured through the process of transmuting internalization, in which selfobject functions are taken over by the child, therby rendering the actual presence of the selfobject less vital or even unnecessary. For example, comforting selfobject experiences eventually enable the child to self-soothe and to regulate his or her self-esteem under the impact of stress, criticism, or disappointments.

Kohut uses the term "optimal frustration" to explain how these transmuting internalizations form. In the context of the selfobject's empathic responsiveness to the child, transient and minor frustrations normally occur that enable the child to "take in" what was previously done for him or her. The child internalizes the selfobject's functions and characteristics in an individualized rather than in an identical way, however, using the selfobject environment to foster its own innate potentialities. An example of transmuting internalization via optimal frustration can be seen at times when a mother who sings to her child at bedtime withdraws prior to the child's falling asleep. If this change is timed correctly, and thus is not too traumatic, the child may soothe himself or herself through singing, playing, or talking, thereby identifying with and taking over the mother's function (White & Weiner, 1986). Frustrations that are too abrupt, ongoing, ill-timed, or characteristic of chronic unattunement or lack of empathy with the child's needs interfere with transmuting internalizations and self-cohesion.

Nuclear and Cohesive Self

The infant is born with rudimentary potentialities that form the basis of the core nuclear self. The parents' selective mirroring (approving and confirming) responses to the child's innate and unique unfolding characteristics and their idealizability enable the nuclear self to crystallize. Gradually the self achieves cohesiveness and stability as an enduring structure through the continuing process of transmuting internalization (Kohut & Wolf, 1978).

Kohut originally described the self as bipolar and as containing three parts: (1) one pole that embodies the child's ambitions and strivings for power and success and that flourishes in response to the mother's mirroring of the child's grandiose-exhibitionistic fantasies and behavior, from approximately ages 2 to 4 years; (2) a second pole that reflects the child's idealized goals that develop in empathic relationships with idealizable selfobjects, from about ages 4 to 6; and (3) an intermediate area of basic talents and skills that interact with the "tension arc" formed by the interaction between the two poles of ambitions and goals (Kohut & Wolf, 1978; White & Weiner, 1986).

A strong cohesive self gives the person a sense of vigor, inner harmony, and self-esteem, but the emergent self may also reflect deficiencies that result in fragmentation, enfeeblement, lack of zest, and problems in self-esteem regulation that are so severe as to constitute a self disorder (Kohut & Wolf, 1978).

The Grandiose Self

Kohut draws attention to a normal phase in the child's development in which the grandiose self asserts itself, and to the importance of the selfobject milieu in responding with pleasure and enthusiasm to, rather than suppressing or discouraging, the child's grandiose-exhibitionistic fantasies and behavior. Responsive selfobjects gradually help the child to tolerate the inevitable blows to his or her omnipotence and to deidealize the formerly all-powerful parents nontraumatically. Thus, the process of transmuting internalization gradually transforms infantile grandiosity into healthy ambitions, values, and stable self-esteem. In contrast, a nonempathic selfobject milieu can lead to fixation of the grandiose self as a regressive defense against premature or extreme disillusionment or disappointment in the self or others. This fixation leaves the individual with an underlying weak and vulnerable self.

Narcissistic Rage as a Disintegration Product

Rejecting classical psychoanalytic theory's conception of the primacy of the drives, self psychology views narcissistic rage as a disintegration product resulting from early selfobject failures. When the child experiences severe and protracted exposure to a lack of parental empathy, the self remains enfeebled. This rage is remobilized later in life when the narcissistic or borderline individual experiences disappointments, rejections, a lack of appreciation, misunderstandings, or even minor criticisms from those upon whom they depend as selfobjects. The narcissistic rage reactions that commonly result in these instances are understandable responses to a lack of selfobject attunement when the self structure is weak and lacks sufficient cohesion.

What others regard as clinical manifestations of an individual's defensive regression to Oedipal and preoedipal sexual or aggressive fantasies and behavior are also viewed as disintegration products resulting from insufficiently met selfobject needs. For example, a child's preoccupation with sexual fantasies or seemingly inappropriate demands for attention may be a consequence of the parents' failure to mirror the child's independence and achievements sufficiently. Thus, the many forms of oral, anal, and phallic preoccupations are disintegration products resulting from selfobject failures rather than indicators of instinctual conflicts.

Compensatory Structures

In Kohut's schema, not all structural defects in the self result in pathology since the child may be able to acquire compensatory structures that strengthen the self. These structures enable the person to make up for or repair deficits in one aspect of the self through successful development of its other facets. Thus, the child has more than one chance to achieve self-cohesion. In contrast to defenses, which cover over enduring defects in the self and are used to improve low self-esteem, compensatory structures actually foster self-cohesiveness.

The Origins of Borderline Pathology

Kohut's writings focus on the development and treatment of narcissistic disorders that he saw as primary disturbances of the self, which were related to but different from the more severe borderline states and psychoses (Kohut & Wolf, 1978). Borderline states reflect a "permanent or protracted" break-up and enfeeblement of the self, which is covered over by rigid defenses that protect the highly vulnerable self from fragmentation (Tolpin, 1980). While the self may collapse if defenses are weakened or tampered with, borderlines generally function at a higher level and remain more reality-oriented than psychotics. In contrast to borderline states, the narcissistic disorders are characterized by the propensity to transient, less severe break-ups in the self, and their defenses are not as rigid or essential as protections against the complete collapse of the self. Thus, unlike the ego psychological and object-relations conceptions of borderline pathology as a stable defensive structure, Kohut sees borderline defenses as reflecting underlying defects in the self stemming from non-gratifying or traumatic experiences with others.

Consistent with his views on self development, Kohut does not specify an exact time for the emergence of borderline states. Presumably the empathic failures of the selfobject milieu for mirroring, idealization, and twinship would have to be fairly pervasive and prolonged so that the child's ability to acquire sufficient compensatory structures and thus, some measure of self-cohesion, is greatly compromised. The borderline often develops schizoid and paranoid attitudes and behavior that ward off the selfobject attachments that would result in overt psychosis. Because of the realistic threat of self-fragmentation, the borderline individual cannot allow himself or herself to become attached to selfobjects or to use them for overcoming weaknesses in the self. In some instances, borderline persons desperately seek intense merger experiences with others in which they attempt to acquire necessary sustenance, but their concomitant fear of fragmentation and inordinate sensitivity to disappointment makes these attachments highly fragile and tumultuous.

Borderline individuals' defects in self structure leave them with a chronic and overwhelming sense of anxiety or dread, and contribute to problems in self-regulation, self-control, self-soothing, low self-esteem, and a sense of personal inadequacy. The absence of sufficient transmuting internalizations results in a search for others to perform archaic selfobject functions and to help maintain themselves against fragmentation. Likewise they frequently abuse drugs, alcohol, and food, and engage in indiscriminate sexuality or other compulsive, dangerous, or exciting activities for similar purposes (Palombo, 1983).

Both building upon and departing somewhat from Kohut's view of borderline pathology as reflecting permanent defects in the self, Brandchaft and Stolorow (1984) argue that borderline pathology is on a continuum with narcissistic disorders. It always is codetermined by the interactions between a vulnerable self and a failing selfobject. Consequently, if the surrounding milieu is able to be empathic with the archaic selfobject needs and defenses of those who show even severe weakness in their self structures, the so-called borderline features will fade, exposing the underlying narcissistic vulnerability.

Underlying this view is a reformulation of what Kernberg and others have labeled as the borderline individual's pathological defenses, such as splitting, projective identification, denial, idealization, and grandiosity. In an earlier writing, Stolorow and Lachmann (1980) make a distinction between mechanisms that reflect defenses related to structural conflict and those that represent an earlier arrest of ego development. In their view, defenses are the end products of developmental lines or sequences and thus, one can identify their prestages. The development of borderline and narcissistic individuals is often stuck at these earlier points, which represent arrests in self-object differentiation and integration, although in other instances it can reflect the higher structural conflict level of development. When individuals are insufficiently structured they seek archaic modes of relating to others. In the treatment relationship this can be misinterpreted as evidence of pathological defenses, often to the detriment of the patient. Instead, the therapist functions to promote the structuralization of precarious self- and object-representations. In a later formulation, which shows more allegiance to self psychology rather than an effort to integrate psychoanalytic ego psychology and self psychology, Brandchaft and Stolorow (1984a, 1984b) point to the developmental arrests in the self that these behaviors represent and the need for the therapist to relate to the patient's behavior empathically thereby espousing hopes for a "resumption of development."

ADLER AND BUIE'S INSUFFICIENT MATERNAL HOLDING EXPERIENCES

Adler (1985) and Buie and Adler (1982) see borderline pathology as reflecting a more identifiable and stable type of developmental deficit than do Brandchaft and Stolorow. Drawing on Piaget (1937), Fraiberg (1969), Sandler and Rosenblatt (1962), Winnicott (1953), Tolpin (1971), Kohut (1971), and Mahler (1975) they trace the developmental process by which the infant acquires the capacity for evocative memory. This ability, which begins at about 18 months of age, enables the child to evoke the memory of an object in the absence of visual cues, and results from mothering that is not good enough earlier than the rapprochement subphase of the separation–individuation process. It is a higher level achievement than the attainment of the capacity for recognition memory that occurs at about 8 months of age. Then the infant is able to recognize an object as familiar in the object's presence. Both of these capacities depend on the maturation of the infant's cognitive functions that make internalized object relations possible, and also on the maternal holding function. The mother's ability to provide reliable soothing and caring enables the child to take in "holding introjects" that stabilize over time.

The capacity for evocative memory is fragile for a time and is easily lost initially if the child undergoes prolonged separation from the mother. Its acquisition permits the child greater autonomy, as the child's ability to remember the mother's presence results in self-soothing capacities. It also enables the child to overcome the devastating sense of aloneness, panic, or depression resulting from separations from significant others.

The core deficit that leads to borderline pathology is the lack of a solid evocative memory in the area of object relations, as a consequence of insufficient maternal holding experiences. Adler and Buie see this deficit in positive introjects as more basic to borderline pathology than the splitting that wards off destruction of the "good" self- and object-representations from the "bad" ones. Splitting implies that the child has acquired "good" internal introjects and occurs later developmentally. Because of Buie and Adler's emphasis on borderline patients' lack of holding introjects rather than their ego pathology per se, Druck (1989), in a recent book, has referred to their approach as reflecting a representational-deficit rather than ego deficit or self-deficit model.

The deficit in the capacity for evocative memory leaves the borderline child, and later the adult, with a terrible sense of aloneness, fears of abandonment, annihilation anxiety, and loss of self-cohesion in the face of separation experiences. Whatever capacity may exist is easily lost under stress, and resultant rage and panic reactions in turn intensify feelings of alienation and aloneness. Borderline individuals also experience a need–fear dilemma in which they simultaneously long for and are threatened by intense closeness with others. The fear prevents the person from entering into or experiencing others as sufficiently holding–soothing and leads to a defensive patterning of interpersonal relationships that obstructs the development of a solid sense of self.

STERN'S FOUR SENSES OF THE SELF

A novel account of the developmental process comes from the work of Daniel Stern (1985), who systematically studied child–mother interactions. Using sophisticated video technology and other observational techniques, Stern was able to trace the complex and subtle interpersonal transactions that form the basis of his theory of self development. While he does not address the origins of borderline or other psychopathology specifically, his developmental concepts have significant clinical implications.

Stern's work represents a major example of the observed infant perspective, which he believes complements the clinical infant perspective. Like Kohut, Stern sees the self as the major organizer of the personality, present in a rudimentary form at birth. In contrast to Kernberg's object-relations and Mahler's separation–individuation theories, both of which describe the newborn infant as going through autistic and symbiotic stages, Stern gives evidence that the infant is born with an innate sense of separateness from others, and that over time the child's self evolves as a consequence of complex interpersonal transactions. He argues that while there are stages in the development of the self as the child's physical and mental maturation propels him or her to face certain adaptive tasks, these stages are not time bound, nor does the individual grow out of any particular phase. Each one becomes a distinct form of experience that gets further elaborated over time as the individual deals with later developmental tasks. For example, the attainment of autonomy is not tied to a particular age but is worked on at various points in the life cycle.

Developmental Concepts

Delineating four phases of self development that he prefers to call "domains of relatedness," Stern (1985) views each domain as codetermined by the growing infant's innate maturational capacities and the nature and degree of attunement of the caretaker environment.

The Sense of Emergent Self

From birth onwards, Stern's infant, like Tolpin's self psychological baby (1986), is an active organism that seems able to process important information about the external and interpersonal world. It can make distinctions between people by smell and sound, identify familiar objects that it has sucked, and make connections between stimuli based on their intensity. The infant quickly engages in behavior that confirms its own existence as a separate being and builds up a stable picture of the physical characteristics of the interpersonal milieu.

The Sense of Core Self

As early as 2 to 3 months and continuing until about 7 months, the infant forms an organized sense of a core self that has two aspects: the first, in which the infant acquires a clear grasp of both its own and the significant other's separate physical presence; and the second, in which it achieves a sense of the mutual influence that exists between itself and another. This view contrasts sharply with that of Mahler, who describes this period as a symbiotic one. In fact, Stern argues strongly that the infant's ability to merge with the mother is a product of its separateness rather than a reflection of a normal symbiotic phase.

The infant's sense of a core self as separate from the other is composed of four factors that become integrated: (1) self-agency — owning one's actions and not owning the actions of others; (2) self-coherence — being a physical whole with boundaries and a center of action; (3) self-affectivity — experiencing patterned inner qualities of feelings; and (4) self-history — having a sense of continuity (Stern, 1985). The infant's sense of its core self in relation to the other is contingent upon satisfying episodes of mutual regulation that build up over time. Primary or secondary merger experiences in which the infant is undifferentiated from the other because of either its lack of boundaries or the loss of those that are tenuous, occur. Gratifying experiences, in which the mother–infant dyad both cue and respond to one another as separate beings who influence but do not obliterate one another, are essential to the firming up of the sense of core self.

The Sense of Subjective Self

Between 7 and 9 months the infant moves beyond experiencing itself and others in terms of physical characteristics and discovers inner mental qualities. For example, the child not only reacts positively to the mother's overt comforting or empathic behavior but recognizes her empathic process. Likewise, the child's awareness of his or her own and others' intentions and affects permits an intersubjective relatedness to develop. This period marks the beginning of the child's capacity for true intimacy and sharing of experience.

The child's attainment of a sense of subjective self builds upon but does not supersede or replace the sense of a core self, which continues to expand. Unlike Mahler, who describes the child's differentiation from the mother at this time, Stern draws attention to the child's growing ability to share with the mother during this period. In fact, he criticizes earlier ego psychological views for their over-emphasis on separation–individuation and neglect of the beginnings of intersubjective relatedness.

The Sense of Verbal Self

At about 15 to 18 months the child begins to acquire the capacity for language and symbolization. The attainment of this verbal domain of relatedness adds a different dimension to the way the child experiences himself or herself, others, and the world. The child becomes capable of viewing himself or herself objectively, performing empathic acts, engaging in symbolic play, and thinking. Language not only facilitates separation–individuation but also helps to unite two persons in a common use of symbols.

Clinical Implications

Stern's work does not address adult psychopathology per se, but instead focuses on the degree of optimal or deviant development of the child's four senses of the self. It is not yet clear which of the deviations that he observed are linked to later clinical disorders. Those that were identified in the subjects he studied, however, always reflected mismatching or unattuned transactions between the child and his or her caretaker, rather than residing in the infant alone. Constitutional or genetic factors seemed to contribute greatly to the different ways infants interacted with the world, but the mother's ability to fit herself to the child's temperament, needs, and behavioral patterns was also crucial in the development of the four domains of relatedness.

Since there are formative periods for each sense of self, it is likely that these are sensitive times with respect to later functioning. It is also likely, however, that certain disorders arise as a consequence of misattunement in all domains of relatedness, rather than being linked to one in particular. For example, the borderline individual's problems in self-cohesion described by Kohut may arise from mismatching at many levels of self development rather than those at one stage alone.

CONCLUSION

This summary of major developmental concepts shows the richness and diversity of theories regarding both personality formation and the origins of borderline disorders. While pointing to the significance of the infant–caretakers interactions in borderline development, the theories differ with respect to: the nature–nurture controversy; whether borderline pathology is stage-specific; whether it reflects object relations, ego, or self pathology; its degree of stability; and its precise dynamic and structural pathology. Research paradigms that can be used to help validate developmental concepts and theories are necessary (Glassman, 1988). Likewise, efforts to integrate the clinical infant and observed infant perspectives through longitudinal studies of early childhood patterns and later psychopathology may help to clarify the clinical relevance of these disparate formulations. The varying developmental hypotheses that have been presented in this chapter have different clinical implications, which will be discussed in more detail later in the book.

5

Family Characteristics
and Dynamics

In contrast to the psychodynamic perspectives on development that were described in Chapter 4, family-oriented theorists view both the family of origin and current interpersonal interactions as generating and sometimes perpetuating borderline pathology. They have attempted to describe the characteristics and dynamics found in families and couples in which there is at least one borderline member. Most of the data about so-called borderline families and couples are drawn from the clinical situation, in which therapists either reconstruct a picture of the parental personalities and family life based on what is reported, or from direct observations of family interactions during the treatment process. Some clinical researchers have attempted to use quantitative research techniques in their study of such families. These combined efforts, however, have delineated different patterns and lend themselves to varied interpretations. This chapter will consider the main contributors to this approach.

WOLBERG'S CLINICAL OBSERVATIONS

Basically a psychodynamically-oriented clinician who worked with individuals, Wolberg nevertheless became quite interested in the impact of past parental personalities on the development of borderline pathology, although she did not address the need for family treatment per se. Summarizing her earlier clinical observations, Wolberg (1982) classifies the mothers of her borderline patients as: (1) obsessive-compulsive; (2) self-oriented, competitive, and masculine; (3) paranoid; or (4) passive and schizoid. Fathers she characterized as: (1) passive-aggressive; (2) hostile, aggressive, attacking, and controlling; (3) paranoid; and (4) mildly psychopathic, promoting antisocial behavior. Building on Freud's view of oedipal dynamics, she proposes a model of triadic sadomasochistic relations among parents and children that are associated with borderline development. In the first of the two patterns of triadic relations that cause borderline pathology, the father rejects the son and pushes him toward the mother, who, in turn, pits him against the father due to her hostility toward men. The son, who needs the father, identifies with him and takes on his hostility. His unconscious hatred for the father is accompanied by guilt, and his relationship with the mother, with whom he also identifies, is ambivalent but more kindly. In the second pattern, it is the mother who rejects the daughter and pushes her toward the father. He, in turn, pits her against the mother due to his hostility toward women. A similar pattern to the one described in the first instance then ensues. Thus, Wolberg views the rejection of a particular child by both parents as a key factor in the development of borderline pathology. In her descriptions of family life one can identify a type of triangulation whereby a child becomes embroiled in the marital struggle.

Wolberg was among the first clinicians to draw attention to the importance of projective mechanisms in borderline families. She found that parents tend to use a particular child in the service of their own defenses when they feel anxious. The child, in turn, protects himself or herself by identifying with the aggressor, and takes on what has been projected onto him or her.

SHAPIRO AND COLLEAGUES' INTENSIVE CLINICAL STUDIES

Based on their intensive clinical studies of 40 families of hospitalized borderline adolescents at the National Institute of Mental Health, Shapiro, Zinner, Shapiro, and Berkowitz (1975), Shapiro, Shapiro, Zinner, and Berkowitz (1977), and Zinner and Shapiro (1972, 1975) describe what they feel to be the main characteristics of borderline families. Integrating family systems thinking with ego psychology and object-relations theory, they link early family life to borderline development. The majority of the families they observed showed a pattern of overinvolvement and enmeshment although some were rejecting. In their view, both parents of a potential borderline individual suffer from unresolved separation–individuation issues in their families of origin, resulting in conflicts over *autonomy* or *dependency* that are "put into" their relationships with a particular child through the mechanism of projective identification. During the separation–individuation stages of this offspring's childhood and adolescence the family undergoes a regression in which the intense anxiety of the parents, who are not necessarily borderline themselves, mobilizes primitive defensive operations, including splitting, projective identification, and denial. Qualities of "goodness" or "badness" are invested in different members of the family so that each seems one-dimensional (all loving and accepting or all rejecting and punishing). Marital defenses are complementary and lead to collusive interactions. Those parents who deny their own autonomous wishes, which are associated with "badness," are threatened by and resist their children's moves toward increased autonomy. They are unable to support their child's or adolescent's autonomous behavior without fearing the rupture of positive family relationships. In contrast, those parents who deny their own dependent strivings that are associated with "badness," are intolerant of their children's appropriate dependent needs and cannot provide a nurturing holding environment. The parents' projections of their disavowed or "split off" needs onto a particular child, who stimulates their unresolved pathology, compel the child to comply with what has been projected in order to allay his or her anxiety. The offspring's ego functioning and ability to evolve and consolidate a separate and whole identity or self are affected.

In describing the dynamics of those families where there is more overt narcissistic pathology, Berkowitz et al. (1974) note the parents' lack of adequate psychic structure in the area of self-esteem regulation. They tend to vacillate between haughty, grandiose, and controlling behavior and feelings of weakness, powerlessness, and inadequacy, to be over-dependent on others' approval, and to be extremely sensitive to criticism or the absence of praise. They relate to their offspring as representatives of an earlier object from whom they have not separated, and use them as narcissistic supports to bolster their self-esteem. Their childrens' moves toward separation are experienced as injuries and threats to self-esteem. The child complies with parental needs in order to allay anxiety and prevent the parents' rage.

Concurring with Shapiro and his group's views of the role of projective identification and splitting in families of borderline individuals, Schwoeri and Schwoeri (1981, 1982) observe that parentification or the reversal of parent-child roles are prevalent in such families, along with diffuse generational boundaries, the bland acceptance of violence among family members, and the absence of parental rules and discipline. They regard much of the borderline individual's anger and acting-out as an attempt to deal with fears of the perceived threat of parental disapproval and abandonment. The child's attempts to reject the obligations and intense loyalty that are expected of him or her result in guilt and depression.

The following two case vignettes illustrate how the mechanisms of splitting and projective identification, as well as problems around autonomy and dependence, show themselves in the families of borderline patients.

Debbie, age 18, lived with her parents, the Fines, who were both psychiatrists in an affluent suburb. Debbie's older brother, who was the parents' favorite child, lived at college. In her last year of high school Debbie became increasingly withdrawn, depressed, suicidal, and self-mutilating. When her mother discovered cuts that Debbie had made on her arms, the parents reluctantly sought help for Debbie from a well-known psychiatrist, who became alarmed by her suicidal intent and admitted her to a hospital. Debbie saw herself as a total failure and blamed herself for her problems. She described her parents as wonderful and herself as unattractive, inadequate, and socially backward. She felt different from her peers and was quite dependent on her parents for companionship, which they provided reluctantly and resentfully. They found her depression draining and her company boring. They urged her to socialize with friends and were intolerant of her complaining and clinging behavior. Comparing Debbie unfavorably to their son, the parents could not understand Debbie's inability to "grow up" as she had the benefit of all the material and emotional advantages that they did not have as children.

Each parent had come from poor, immigrant families in which they were the oldest of numerous children and were expected to raise themselves. Each parent had a miserable childhood and suffered neglect and physical abuse at times. Extremely intelligent and hard-working, they put themselves through college and medical school with the help of scholarships and loans. When they married in their late 20s they had achieved what looked like a "perfect" life financially, professionally, and socially. "We vowed to put our unhappy childhoods behind us." They cultivated the interests, values, and manners of economically affluent people. Highly independent, they prided themselves on having "pulled themselves up by the bootstraps" without any help from their own families of origin, and tried to be generous and "good" parents. Their first child, Alex, was easy to raise, and his appeal and talent attracted positive attention from others. This was a source of esteem to the parents.

Debbie was more of a problem from birth. She was sickly, always "hungry," and made the mother feel inadequate. She also resembled her maternal grandmother, which was source of dismay to her mother. When Alex was 5 and Debbie was 2 the mother returned to full-time private practice and hired a live-in housekeeper to take care of the children. Debbie remembers being extremely lonely. She was allowed to call her mother in the 10-minute intervals between patients but always felt she was being a "pest" if she did so. She learned that the only way to get her parents' attention was to have problems, and so had an abundance of difficulties in school. Her parents often teased her for being "babyish" when she sought their affection and approval or when she cried after fights with her brother, who often hurt her physically. She was a mediocre student and would be reduced to tears easily if she felt criticized or rejected. Despite the Fines' dedication to helping others with emotional problems, they were tightly controlled in their expression of feelings. While they had a busy professional and social life, they rarely spent time together alone. They denied having overt conflicts and seldom showed strong emotions to one another. Neither anger nor any other intense display of feeling was a part of their way of communicating with one another. Debbie was more emotional. According to the parents, any anger they experienced resulted from Debbie's behavior. Both the Fines and Debbie seemed to agree that she was the problem in the family. She was "the bad seed" in the sense that she embodied many of the characteristics that her parents attempted to deny in themselves—for example, their dependency, weakness, low self-esteem, emotionality, and especially their anger and depression. They were "good" and they maintained their compensatory sense of perfection by repudiating any qualities that were associated with "badness." Alex, their first-born, carried their "goodness" while Debbie embodied the "badness" that the parents hated but simultaneously needed to express through her. She was exposing their inadequacies. Debbie was trapped and unable either to individuate and develop her own self or to remain in her depreciated, depressed, and dysfunctional but necessary role.

Anthony, age 16, was hospitalized briefly when one of his high school teachers advised his parents, Mr. and Mrs. Bork, that he was abusing drugs and alcohol and was a serious candidate for a drug overdose. Humiliated, angry, and panicky, the parents consulted their family physician who became fearful and arranged for the admission. The episode that triggered the teacher's concern involved Anthony's having confided in him that he had been driving after smoking marijuana and drinking. Anthony became enraged at his parents after a few days in the hospital for "putting me here and ruining my life" and persuaded his psychiatrist to discharge him. He and the Borks were referred for family treatment.

This incident followed a period of great tumult in the Bork household. In sessions, the parents recited a litany of Anthony's difficulties: He no longer wanted to eat dinner with them; he refused to comply with the curfew that they set; he was failing courses because he never studied; he talked back to them and used foul language; he spent more time out of the house than in it; he acted as if he were a guest in the family who did not have any responsibilities; he always asked for money but would never discuss how he spent what he had been given; he never cut his hair and wore clothes that made him look terrible; and he showed no interest in acting like a "civilized human being." His father called him "a bum," engaged in lengthy tirades, and was sometimes on the verge of physically attacking Anthony, while his mother attempted to control almost every aspect of his behavior, including what he ate. Both parents fought about how to deal with him. The mother accused her husband of siding with Anthony against her, which he did at times when he thought his wife was being too harsh and controlling. She thought he was overidentifying with Anthony, who acted "irresponsibly" in ways that her husband had. She was most concerned about Anthony's school problems and his not helping her with chores. Mrs. Bork also attempted to protect Anthony from her husband's escalating rage when his son would come home an hour late for dinner, wearing clothes that were distinctively "punk." More than once Anthony had broken a window or hurt his hand when angry. Mr. Bork drank, and Mrs. Bork worked long hours and compulsively cleaned her house in order to escape the family conflict. Mrs. Bork was furious that her husband loafed and drank while she did the chores, and Mr. Bork was resentful that his wife never spent time with him. Anthony and his parents were out of control, and mutual accusations filled their home life. Despite their conflicts with Anthony, however, Mrs. Bork continued to wake him up every morning and bring him his breakfast and Mr. Bork bought expensive presents for him.

The parents indicated to the therapist that they fought from the beginning of their marriage. While considering divorce several times, they remained together. Each used Anthony as a companion and confidant at times and scapegoated him at others. Assertive and stubborn from an early age, Anthony resisted parental efforts to make him conform. Both wanted him to be compliant, dependent, and dutiful as they were being with one another and as their parents had expected them to be. Both had rebelled against their families of origin, which had been very suffocating, but also felt that they had disappointed their parents, were guilty about their breaking away, and suffered from chronic feelings of unworthiness behind their facade of competence. Despite their overt unhappiness with Anthony, Mr. and Mrs. Bork sabotaged Anthony's healthier efforts at individuation, which they equated with their own "badness" and which also threatened their relationship equilibrium.

GRINKER AND ASSOCIATES' QUANTITATIVE STUDY

The first clinicians to attempt to delineate the family characteristics of borderline patients more systematically, Grinker, Werble, and Drye (1968) studied the families of 47 nonschizophrenic patients that were classified as borderline. A 69-item checklist of family traits was rated for each family on the basis of data collected in a routine social work evaluation at Michael Reese Hospital in Chicago. The research identified three types of families: Type I—those that were not a mutually protective unit; Type II—those that were excessively protective; and Type III—those who denied problems.

The 19 families in Type I showed chronic and overt marital and family conflict, discord, and competition; rejecting and negative attitudes and affect in the mother–child relationships; rejection or conflict about parenthood itself, and confused communication. Type II contained six cases which were characterized by overinvolvement and intrusiveness, a resisting of the separation of the patient from the family, and a submerging of the self-identity of the child. The nine families in Type III showed a denial of family problems, mixed affects, and a submergence of the self-identity of the child.

WALSH'S CHECKLIST STUDY

In her Chicago study of 14 hospitalized nonschizophrenic cases that were considered to be borderline, Walsh (1977) developed a checklist of separation stress events and a family relationships checklist that were scored on the basis of patient reports. The nine female and five male subjects were primarily single, in their 20s, and came from middle-class families. Eight were Jewish with the six remaining cases divided between Protestant and Catholic.

Only six of the fourteen patients came from intact families, reflecting a significantly higher percentage of parent loss than was found in a comparison group of 80 schizophrenic patients. In over half of the cases there was serious parental physical and/or mental illness. In 13 cases the patients reported the onset of their symptoms shortly after they tried to separate from their families. Walsh concludes that these borderline families showed patterns of unrelatedness, neglect, negative and conflictual relationships, overt hostility and rejection, and sometimes frank physical or sexual abuse. This finding seems somewhat at odds, however, with her observation that eight of the patients reported overinvolvement with at least one parent, and feelings of being controlled, made overdependent, and obligated to comply with rigid, unrealistic parental expectations.

GUNDERSON AND COLLEAGUES' COMPARATIVE RESEARCH

Gunderson, Kerr, and Englund (1980) are the only investigators who conducted a comparative study of the family characteristics of three in-patient groups in Boston: 12 patients with borderline personality disorder using Gunderson's criteria, 12 patients with paranoid schizophrenia, and 12 patients with neurotic disturbances. They sought to determine whether the families of borderline patients could be distinguished from the families of other types of patients. Using extensive family evaluations that were obtained routinely as part of the patients' treatment, two raters evaluated all the study cases on 72 family traits that were divided into 11-item groups reflecting more general characteristics. The eight female and the four male borderline patients showed a mean age of 17.5 years.

The items that differentiated the borderline families from the other groups were: maternal psychosis; poor enforcement of rules; absence of maternal overinvolvement with the identified patient; and a tendency for one child to be viewed as "good" and another seen as "bad." The parents' marriages were characterized by a tight marital bond that excluded the child, and an absence of a maternal eroticized relationship with the child who became borderline. Both parents and the siblings reflected greater pathology than in the other groups, and the mothers were less likely to turn to the borderline child for gratification.

These researchers conclude that the main features of borderline families are a consistent pattern of neglect and underinvolvement, severe parental pathology, and a rigid marital bond at the expense of the patient, with little overt hostility. The study's findings are consistent with Shapiro and his associates' view that parental reliance on projective mechanisms and denial is significant in borderline families, but not with their conclusion that the parents were highly overinvolved and tended to oppose their childrens' separation–individuation. In fact, the parents in the Gunderson, Kerr, and Englund study generally experienced their children as too dependent on them and wanted to distance from them. The authors take the view that parent–child difficulties become more intense when their borderline offsprings' ego deficits are unmasked, usually in adolescence when there are greater demands for autonomous functioning. The increased neediness in the borderline adolescent, who has previously adapted to parental unavailability and unrelatedness, is met with nonconstructive parental responses. The writers do acknowledge, however, that their clinical experience shows that there is a minority of borderline families that manifest the overinvolvement pattern and for whom the adolescent's growing independence rather than continued dependency is threatening.

GOLDSTEIN'S THREE FAMILY TYPES

In a paper presented in 1981 at the 58th Annual Meeting of the American Orthopsychiatric Association in New York, Goldstein reported the findings of her study of the families of 28 borderline cases hospitalized at either New York State Psychiatric Institute or New York Hospital, Cornell Medical Center, Westchester Division. The patients were diagnosed using both Kernberg's structural interview approach (1977) and Gunderson's Diagnostic Interview for Borderlines (Gunderson, Kolb, & Austin, 1981) as part of a more extensive research project (Kernberg et al., 1981). Checklists were developed to evaluate the families in four main areas: (1) parental attitudes toward the identified patient; (2) the nature of parent–child relationships; (3) the nature of family conflict; and (4) the nature of the parents' marital relationship. Two research assistants rated the checklists on the basis of transcripts of research interviews with the parents, the social worker's routine written psychosocial assessment of the family, and the primary therapist's written evaluation of the identified patient.

The mean age of the patients was 24, and there were 20 females and 8 males. Almost all were single. The families came from middle-class socioeconomic strata and generally were college educated. Over 50% of the cases were Jewish and the rest were equally divided among Protestant and Catholic. Only slightly more than half (57%) of the families were intact, as compared to 68% in a comparable group of families of schizophrenic patients, a finding corresponding to that reported by Walsh. These families also experienced multiple external stresses due to employment problems, financial instability or dependency, career pressures, physical or mental illness, geographic changes, and nonsupportive extended family relationships during the early childrearing years.

In almost all of the cases the parents viewed the borderline patient as special in either a "good" or "bad" way from birth. In describing their children the parents typically used such expressions as "chip off the old block" or adjectives such as most gifted, talented, intelligent, compliant, independent, needy, demanding, difficult, different, attractive, or aggressive. While in many instances the parents retained this view of the patient, in others they expressed disappointment and anger that the patient had "turned out" this way.

The checklist evaluation identified three family types: the overinvolved family (12 cases); the rejecting family (11 cases); and the idealizing or denying family (5 cases). A profile of the characteristics of each type of family follows.

Profile I: The Enmeshed or Overinvolved Family

The overinvolved families showed intense, overt hostility and conflict in which the patient was triangulated. The families seemed highly enmeshed. One parent often was idealizing, needy, and overprotective of the patient while the other was devaluing, aloof, and rejecting. Sometimes the parents reversed these polar attitudes. Quite controlling, the parents generally experienced difficulty in separating from the patient. They were very willing to be involved in the treatment process when the patient was hospitalized. The following case vignette illustrates these patterns.

Martin, an 18-year-old high school senior, was admitted to the hospital after taking an overdose of sleeping pills. His parents, Mr. and Mrs. Robbins, found him after becoming concerned that he had slept through dinner. They broke down the locked door to his room and took him to a nearby hospital, where he had been admitted briefly several months earlier after threatening to kill himself. Martin began to see a private psychiatrist after discharge but eventually dropped out of treatment. Mr. and Mrs. Robbins were quite worried about Martin, who was failing academically and who frequently drank to the point of intoxication. They felt impotent in controlling his behavior and fought with him constantly, as well as with one another about how to best deal with him. When they found him unconscious, their worst fears had come to pass. They agreed to admit Martin to the hospital but were unprepared for the separation from him, and soon became angry and panicky as a result of the unit's no visiting policy. They described their separation from Martin as "an amputation" and telephoned Martin several times a day. While seeing the social worker weekly, they called her and the doctor frequently. In sessions they alternately blamed Martin, one another, and themselves for Martin's problems.

An only child, Martin appeared especially fragile at birth. Both parents were chronic worriers about all aspects of his behavior — for example, they were frightened that sand would get in his eyes when he played at the beach as a child; they were concerned that other children would beat him up when he was going to school; and they were nervous about his riding subways and buses. While describing their marriage as loving, both parents fought bitterly about sex, money, Martin, in-laws, friends, leisure-time, and so on. These fights were chronic and occurred almost every night at the dinner table. Their disputes about Martin were particularly volatile. Mrs. Robbins described herself as very "overprotective" and a "tough disciplinarian." At the same time she was angry at Martin for being so weak and at her husband for being too "easy" with him. Mr. Robbins described himself as "babying" Martin and letting him get his way, but was also angry at Martin for not "acting his age" and for his passivity and lack of aggressiveness. Mr. Robbins accused his wife of making Martin into a homosexual by hugging and kissing him but also complained that Martin was not affectionate enough with him. Mrs. Robbins felt that her husband treated Martin like "a little girl" and did not know how to be a father. Both parents looked to their son for companionship and affection but complained that the other was doting on and infantilizing him. The parents had never thought of separation or divorce, indicating that they could not live without one another and were "old-fashioned" about marriage.

Profile II: The Alienated or Rejecting Family

The rejecting families each viewed the patient as different, unwelcome, "bad," or an "enemy." The parents believed that family life would be peaceful if the patient would not disrupt it. They sought distance from the patient or typically hoped that the treatment would help the patient to control his or her behavior. The patient may have been highly valued at one time, but somehow had disappointed or frustrated the parents. The parents did not acknowledge marital difficulties and seemed to have a tight bond that excluded the patient. Any marital discord was blamed on the patient. The parents often seemed satisfied with little contact with the patient during hospitalization, and were reluctant to be involved more than minimally in the treatment process. The following example shows these characteristics.

Joan, a single, 27-year-old animal research assistant, was admitted to the hospital for long-term treatment after a history of substance abuse, repeated short-term hospitalizations following suicide attempts, and several years of intermittent private psychotherapy. She had miraculously survived her last suicide attempt in which she jumped from an open window. Joan's parents, Mr. and Mrs. Dinkins, were pessimistic about her chances for becoming a "normal" person. While they were "horrified" and "shocked" at her most recent suicide attempt, they were "fed up" with Joan's inability "to pull her life together" and with her difficulties "in standing on her own two feet." They felt estranged from her since she went to college, but had never felt close to her even before that. She was always a particularly "demanding" child who never seemed satisfied or happy. Stubborn and temperamental, she was "difficult" to understand and never was "lovable." Mr. and Mrs. Dinkins also never liked Joan's friends, who seemed to be "losers."

Both parents viewed Joan as quite intelligent and gifted but doubted that she would ever do anything with her life. They tried to give her advice and to do things for her when she was growing up but felt totally unappreciated and exploited. They wished she would have the incentive to get better and to become self-reliant rather than expect them to help her. The parents described their 29-year marriage as quite satisfying and relatively problem free except for the burden of Joan's difficulties. Very compatible, unlike other couples they knew, they thought that Joan was jealous of their relationship because she would say things like "Why don't you fight?" or "You get along too well." Joan lived at home intermittently since college and the parents reported feeling better when she was away. During the hospitalization neither parent experienced difficulty with the separation from Joan. In fact, they seemed relieved at not seeing her. They rarely called and kept in contact through letters. They were willing to help out financially but were resistant to regular contact with the social worker or doctor. They called from time to time to find out how Joan was progressing.

Profile III: The Idealizing or Denying Family

In the idealizing or denying families the parents and the patient saw one another as nearly "perfect" and minimized the seriousness of the patient's difficulties. The either regarded the patient's hospitalization as an alternative to college dormitory life, or wished to take the patient home quickly despite his or her severe suicidal or other self-destructive behavior. Presenting a picture of complete harmony, the parents could not admit to family or marital conflict. While giving lip service to the importance of their being included in the treatment process, the parents resisted any suggestions that they were a part of the problem. If therapists confronted their denial, they were perceived as "enemies" who were destroying family life. The following case example shows these features.

Since graduating from college, Dina, a single, 27-year-old copy editor, was hospitalized briefly five times in five years for bouts of anorexia, wrist-cutting, and suicide attempts. During high school and college and between hospitalizations she was in private psychotherapy with a number of psychiatrists who were selected and paid by her parents, Mr. and Mrs. Frank. Each time she criticized her therapy to her parents they encouraged her to leave treatment. Dina had to take a leave of absence from college in her second year because of her anorexia. She went down to 71 pounds at that time. Despite Dina's long history of serious emotional difficulties and psychiatric treatment, which dated back to age thirteen, her parents were always shocked when she attempted suicide. While her wrist-slashing attempts were "superficial," on one occasion she went into a coma from an overdose.

The Franks viewed Dina as a very loving and creative child with a kindly disposition, and as someone who had strong values and set high standards for herself. They saw her as especially sensitive to rejection or disappointment but never as having serious emotional problems. Always wanting the "best" for Dina, the parents sought out psychiatrists with excellent credentials as one might search for the right finishing school. Disappointed in the doctors who treated Dina, they saw them as cold, unappreciative of her talents, and insensitive to their own needs. They resented doctors' insinuations that Dina was angry at them and that they needed help in seeing their daughter more realistically. When long-term hospitalization was urged by the last psychiatrist, the Franks were devastated and reluctantly agreed to the recommendation. They hoped that hospitalization would enable Dina "to have more confidence" and "to develop her potential." They felt that she could be doing more to help herself since "our daughter can do anything she wants if she puts her mind to it." The Franks described their family relationships as very happy except when Dina was distressed. They acknowledged shielding Dina somewhat over the years but then commented, "Don't all parents do that?" Optimistic that Dina would "come out of this stage" eventually, they were willing to participate in Dina's treatment. They mainly wanted information about Dina's progress, however, rather than to be included in family sessions, and were very concerned about the effect on Dina of the other "sicker" patients on the unit. They sought continual reassurance that Dina would not be exposed to negative influences.

These family profiles show points of similarity to and differences from the other family research discussed in this chapter. In identifying three characteristic patterns rather than one main constellation in the families of borderline patients, the Goldstein study closely resembles that of Grinker and his colleagues. It is noteworthy that Goldstein found both the overinvolvement pattern observed by Shapiro and his associates and the rejection pattern identified by Gunderson, Kerr, and Englund and Walsh to be present in the borderline families.

These three family patterns also can be explained dynamically in terms of the parental defenses of splitting, denial, projective identification, and need to preserve their narcissistic equilibrium, following Shapiro and his co-workers' views (Goldstein, 1983). Thus, a child who is regarded as "special" at birth (and even earlier in fantasy) becomes a selfobject for one or both of the parents. The child must mirror the parents and conform to parental needs and perceptions. Despite the parents' ability to be "loving" when the child fulfills the part that he or she is assigned, there is a *failure in empathy* with the "whole" child. The family cannot acknowledge the youngster as a separate and distinct person. Attempts to control the child followed by narcissistic rage and rejection when he or she breaks out of or fails to meet parental needs are common. Actual rather than fantasized expulsion from the family may be the cost of the child's becoming his or her own person. The child who is unable to or fails to perform a needed selfobject function from the beginning may become a focus of rejecting and punitive attitudes that become internalized. Children grow up feeling unloved and unlovable. They lack self-esteem and self-cohesion, show conflicts around autonomy and dependence, do not trust their own inner experience, and show deficiencies in ego functioning.

A HISTORY OF SEXUAL ABUSE

An important feature of family life is the presence of sexual abuse. As a more accurate picture of the incidence and prevalence of sexual abuse has developed, it has become increasingly clear that a large number of so-called borderline individuals reflect a history of such incidents. Kroll (1988) suggests that one of the main pathways to the development of borderline disorders is through the repeated experience of sexual abuse, and that histories of both physical and sexual abuse are found commonly in those borderline patients who show brief psychotic episodes. One recent study reported that a history of physical and sexual abuse was found more often in borderline versus non-borderline patients (Herman et al., 1989) and another concluded that female incest victims showed a significantly higher incidence of borderline, avoidant, schizoid, and passive–aggressive pathology, along with anxiety and depression, alcohol abuse, psychotic episodes, and somatic complaints than did non-incest victims (Wheeler & Walton, 1987).

PERSPECTIVES ON COUPLE DYNAMICS

Instead of focusing on the borderline individual's family of origin, a number of theorists have attempted to describe the current interaction of borderline couples.

An Object-Relations Perspective

An object-relations approach to understanding couples (Scharff & Scharff, 1987; Slipp, 1988; Stewart et al., 1975) sees each partner as bringing their problems in internalized object relations into the marriage or partnership. Scripts of the past dominate present interactions, and problems in ego functioning are present. Each member of the couple verbalizes a wish for help, but seems invested in maintaining the marital system and resists change. This leads to chronic marital disharmony, often punctuated by frequent attempts to end the relationship or by other impulsive behaviors. The partners are unhappy with each other but cannot seem to separate or resolve their difficulties. A pattern of intense merging followed by distancing is common. The stalemate that develops reflects each member's unconscious efforts to repair his or her early deficits in the relationship, which unfortunately embodies the original pathology and becomes a fixed, dysfunctional system.

Like the Shapiro group mentioned earlier in this chapter, object-relations couple therapists emphasize the mechanisms of splitting, denial, projective identification, and collusion (Siegel, in press; Stewart et al., 1975). The following describe the individual defenses: splitting refers to the active separation of two contradictory ego states, such as love and hate or qualities of "goodness" or "badness" in order to preserve the illusion of an all "good" self or object; denial enables a person to fail to recognize or accept the presence of an unfavorable characteristic; and projective identification permits an individual to put a disavowed trait or feeling into someone else who is then treated accordingly. In couple relationships, each partner who utilizes splitting, denial, and projective identification experiences his or her own split off or disavowed traits in the other person. For example, a man who sees himself as a victim and does not acknowledge his own abusive behavior selects a woman who is more overtly victimizing whom he then provokes to be abusive. Sometimes it appears as if one partner in the relationship carries all the "badness" and the other all the "goodness." In other instances the partners exchange roles, but rarely do they ever achieve a more harmonious balance. Another pattern one sees in certain couples is their assumption of all the "good" or idealized qualities so that the marriage seems "perfect" while at the same time splitting off the "bad" qualities onto an offspring. As long as the splitting and projective identification continue in this way, however, neither member of the dyad is forced to confront his or her own "unfavorable" traits.

Collusion further complicates couple relationships. As each partner projects selected split off traits onto his or her mate, the other partner accepts what has been projected and acts in accordance with the projection in a collusive manner. In turn, the person who splits and projects then identifies unconsciously with what has been projected onto the other partner and attempts to control the now projected behavior. For example, a woman who prides herself on never being overtly angry splits off her rage and projects it onto her husband whom she provokes to behave in an extremely aggressive fashion. The wife not only feels consciously upset by his reactions but criticizes the husband for his angry outbursts. Sometimes partners will complain of feeling "set up" to respond in a particular way by their mates, who then disapprove of or punish them for their reactions. A criticism of this formulation is that it can be used to "blame the victim" in a relationship by suggesting that the abused party, for example, has provoked the abuse. The following example illustrates how splitting, projective identification, and collusion present in a couple in treatment for escalating marital difficulties.

By the time they sought help after 5 years of marriage, Dave and Barbara could barely speak without screaming at one another. They had separated and reconciled several times during the past year. Seeing her 3-year-old daughter agitated by the couple's near violent fights, Barbara threatened to seek a divorce if Dave would not agree to enter marital treatment. In their first session Barbara bitterly complained, in alternating whiny and sarcastic tones, that Dave was "hypercritical, perfectionist, controlling, selfish, and withholding. All he's interested in is getting 'toys' for himself. He's got to have the newest sports model on the road. He's such a baby. I'm sure he's messing up his business again because he spends all of his time reading car magazines instead of working. If I dare ask him for anything — money, sex, affection, help around the house — I get a 'not now Barbara,' or he withdraws and pouts just to punish me. I'm tired of being treated like 'dirt' and the 'enemy.'" With rapidly escalating and somewhat frightening anger, Dave retorted, "I would treat you better if you would grow up, do what you're supposed to do, and not ask me a hundred times a day to do things that you can take care of yourself. You don't even balance the checkbook yourself, Barbara, so don't give me that shit about how I'm a baby. You conveniently leave out how you can't even handle calling the plumber without asking for my advice. You want to have your cake and eat it too. Grow up! As for my not helping you around the house, you always have to have things done your way. I don't like being controlled." In an exasperated and raised voice Barbara answered, "I don't believe this. *You* don't like being controlled? You're Mr. Control in person. Do you ever tell me how much money we have? I have to come to you like a little girl. Daddy, can I please buy some groceries? Then you tell me that I'm acting like a child. Fuck you." To which Dave responded, "You know, Miss Perfect, you have a 'nasty mouth' and your kid is growing up just like you." Later, in reply to the therapist's request that they describe a time when they got along better, Dave and Barbara each reported cheerfully that they were very compatible and had a lot of fun together. They seemed oblivious to the chronic disharmony in their relationship that they had just been enacting in the session itself. Somewhat ironically, Barbara said that she sometimes thought that Dave had to provoke a fight with her when they were getting along too well.

Further information that was obtained about Dave and Barbara's relationship and personalities supported the following interpretation of their interaction. Both split off and projected onto the other their own "bad" dependent, irresponsible, controlling, and aggressive characteristics. They colluded in alternately assuming the roles of "good" parent and "bad" child. Each felt victimized by the other while splitting off and denying their own victimizing qualities. In the heat of their arguments each totally hated the other, who was viewed as "all bad," and not infrequently their fights led to one or the other leaving the house or threats of violence or divorce. During more peaceful times in the relationship both Dave and Barbara acted as if they were in complete accord and did not acknowledge their difficulties. They felt their relationship was perfect at these times. The couple never were able to attempt to resolve any of their problems. Either they were too intensely embroiled in conflict or they denied their differences altogether. Their relationship took on either "all good" or "all bad" qualities. Further, there was some suggestion that they could not sustain closeness and that their fights followed periods of greater intimacy.

A Self Psychological Perspective

Building on Kohut's view that the need for selfobjects is a lifelong aspect of the human condition, and that self-regard fluctuates with the degree of acceptance and admiration from idealized others, some writers (Schwartzman, 1984; Solomon, 1985; Solomon, 1989) have identified each member of a couple's failure to acknowledge and gratify the partner's selfobject needs as a cause of marital or couple problems. While each partner's need for the other to serve selfobject functions may be considered to be a normal part of close relationships, it is more urgent and complex when individuals suffer from self disorders of a borderline or narcissistic variety. These individuals tend to live out their earlier unfulfilled parental relationships quite dramatically when they couple. They develop "relationships in which the purpose becomes joining together for the perpetuation of fantasies of wholeness, total acceptance, and approval" (Solomon, 1985, p. 144). Frustrated past experiences are alive in the present and selfobject needs are more intense and archaic. When these needs are not met as a consequence of one or both partners failing to function as a mirroring or idealizing selfobject for the other, rage, depressive reactions, injured self-esteem, and fragmentation of the self may result (White, 1984). "Each partner demands change in the other in order to repair damage to the self" (Solomon, 1985, p. 144). Defensive structures appear in both members of a couple when their self-esteem or self-cohesion are endangered that contribute to couple disharmony. Sometimes fighting itself can be a means for maintaining a sense of connection or creating needed distance (Magdoff & Greenberg, 1988).

While both narcissistic and borderline individuals urgently seek to get their partners to meet their archaic selfobject needs, they manifest somewhat different types of needs and responses to selfobject failures. Solomon (1985) suggests that those individuals on the more narcissistic end of the spectrum tend to seek fusion or sameness with their partners and have difficulty tolerating any degree of difference. In contrast, she argues that borderline individuals are more caught in a conflict between their wishes for autonomy and their fears of disapproval or rejection. This distinction, however, may not always be evident and other differences may exist. Adler (1985) argues that the narcissistic individual is more sensitive to blows to self-esteem, while borderline persons fear loss and abandonment. Lachkar (1985) argues that the borderline member of a couple views the narcissist as calming while the narcissist finds the borderline partner's expressiveness exciting. Further, the borderline partner fears abandonment while the narcissist fears being invaded and taken over by the borderline's demands. Frustrating interactive cycles get established. While most writers about borderline disorders describe their alternating merging and distancing behavior, Kohut (1977) emphasizes the borderline's need to protect against fragmentation by avoiding closeness to potential selfobjects, in contrast to the narcissistic individual's need to seek selfobject experiences. The following example shows a couple in conflict stemming from the mutual frustration of selfobject functions.

Angela and Mark were on the verge of breaking up when they desperately sought help as a "last ditch" effort to save their relationship. While dating regularly for 5 years, they had only recently begun living together. Both were creative individuals, and their work often separated them. Mark had numerous brief sexual liaisons with others and Angela had one affair during a period when Mark was involved with someone else. After Mark learned of this relationship he insisted that he and Angela live together, but has never forgiven Angela for her "betrayal" of him. When together they fight bitterly. In their first session, Mark, the more overtly distraught member of the couple, described pliantly how Angela was becoming more and more emotionally and sexually unresponsive to him. He felt that his efforts to show concern and love for Angela were met with aloofness and withdrawal. Her general indifference to him and her rebuffs of his attempts to get her to share her thoughts and feelings with him made him increasingly panicky and explosive. The more he tried to get Angela to respond to him, the more she withheld. On several occasions Mark remorsefully reported, he had lost control and hit Angela. After such an episode he would apologize profusely and they would have a truce for a time until the next escalation. Mark's distress could be stimulated by Angela's brief absences, her criticism of Mark, her voicing of a differing opinion, her wish for some time by herself, her failure to tell Mark the specific details of her daily activities, thoughts, and feelings, or even her talking on the telephone to someone else.

In a somewhat diffident manner, choosing her words very carefully, Angela responded. "Mark won't let me alone. He wants me to be there for him totally when he has the time to notice my existence. He's very possessive and jealous. I am more private with my thoughts and feelings than he is. Maybe it's a problem, but that's how I am. I don't understand why he can't accept that I am not the same as he is. Why does he have to know everything that I do? I need my space. He takes his. He can get so involved in his work that he hardly notices me for days. Can't he understand that I have a life too? I take care of our apartment, cook for him, and help him in his career, not that I always feel like it. Nothing I do is enough." "But darling," Mark said, "I do appreciate you, and that's why I want to be with you." Angela responded "Well, do I always have to want to be with you? For once, it would be nice if you didn't pressure me." Looking deflated, Mark stated, "I just don't think you are attracted to me anymore." Angela retorted "You don't always act in a very attractive way, do you Mark dear?" Mark replied "I really hate when you attack me personally because I don't fit your image." "Well, Mark dear," answered Angela, "I can't help it if you're not my physical type. But there are things you could do to improve yourself. I don't particularly enjoy living with someone who is so disorderly, and you have to admit that some of your personal habits were pretty disgusting when we first got together. If you say you love and appreciate me so much, why can't you take care of yourself better?"

Mark and Angela had achieved a tense but manageable equilibrium prior to their moving in together. Their frequent separations served to regulate their closeness and give them both the space they needed. Mark's involvements with other women kept him from an all encompassing involvement with Angela, who was able to keep Mark in the role of the idealizable but unavailable figure. Their archaic selfobject needs intensified when they began living together and were generally frustrated. Mark sought an intense, undifferentiated, and idealizing relationship with Angela in which she devoted herself to him, shared his every breath, and admired him in order to deal with his fears of abandonment and to regulate his self-esteem. When deprived of her total attention and compliance with his needs he became panicky and felt alone, worthless, and enraged. Frustrated by Angela and unable to soothe himself, he became impulsive and explosive. Caught up in his own feelings, he could not recognize and understand Angela's needs, which, unfortunately, were on a collision course with his. She needed a perfect and idealizable partner who would support her autonomy, make few demands on her, appreciate her efforts, and respect her needs for separateness and space. When Mark repeatedly frustrated her, she became depressed, hypercritical, devaluing, and withholding. She was unable to empathize with Mark's needs and justified her reactions by believing that nothing that she gave Mark would ever be enough. A mutually torturous interaction pervaded their relationship.

CONCLUSION

A family perspective on the development of borderline disorders complements individual psychodynamic explanatory models. The clinical and research findings on family characteristics and dynamics have focused on pathological parental personality traits; primitive defenses such as splitting, denial, and projective identification; conflicts around autonomy and dependence; and the presence of archaic selfobject needs. Differing family patterns have been identified: triadic sadomasochistic relations; overinvolvement and enmeshment; underinvolvement and neglect; rejection; and idealization. Loss, violence, and sexual abuse have been identified in the histories of borderline individuals. Couple dynamics show collusion, distortion, and vicious cycles of mutual frustration stemming from the repetition of early internalized self- and object-representations and archaic selfobject needs. While further investigation is needed regarding whether or not there are particular constellations of borderline families, many theorists agree that past and on-going family transactions play an important role in causing and maintaining borderline pathology.

PART II

CLINICAL THEORY AND TECHNIQUE

6

Conflict-Based
Treatment Models

Chapter 4 discussed the conflict and deficit views of the development of borderline pathology. The treatment implications that stem from these differing perspectives are divergent and even contradictory, although some authors have attempted to put forth a mixed model approach (Chatham, 1985). The two most widely recognized conflict-based treatment models are found in the work of Otto Kernberg (1975, 1984) and James Masterson (1972, 1976) along with his collaborator, Donald Rinsley (1975). This chapter will present and illustrate the main features of their views.

KERNBERG'S EXPRESSIVE PSYCHOTHERAPY

When his views on expressive treatment were evolving Kernberg was influenced by the results of the Psychotherapy Research Project of the Menninger Foundation (Kernberg et al., 1972). This study concluded that those patients with severe ego weakness or borderline conditions improved the most when they received expressive psychotherapy while also undergoing hospitalization at certain points during their clinical course. These findings reinforced Kernberg's growing belief that an intensive treatment aimed at the modification of a borderline patient's core pathology is preferable to a supportive one that focuses only on improving a patient's adaptive functioning.

Treatment Goals and Framework

The goal of expressive psychotherapy with borderline patients is structural change through the modification of pathological defenses and the integration of split part self- and object-representations. Since Kernberg views ego weakness as the product rather than the cause of borderline personality organization, he believes that the ego is strengthened when internalized object-relations pathology is altered. For example, with a patient whose use of splitting diminishes his or her realistic perceptions of others, the therapist's confrontation and interpretation of this defense will improve the patient's capacity for reality testing.

In this treatment model a consistent structure should be established in which: (1) the patient sits up and faces the therapist rather than lies on a couch; (2) the psychotherapy sessions take place a minimum of two times a week, although three weekly meetings are more optimal initially and more frequent sessions may be helpful later; (3) the therapist adheres to a fixed schedule of appointment times for specified intervals and is clear about policies regarding cancellations and missed sessions; (4) the therapist focuses on the patient's current life situation and relationships, particularly early in treatment; (5) the therapist sets limits on the patient's acting-out within the sessions as reflected in extremely provocative or aggressive behavior, demands on the therapist for extra time, personal information, involvement in the patient's life, or need gratification; and (6) the patient's life is sufficiently structured, through hospitalization or other means, so that destructive impulses and behavior are not permitted to disrupt the treatment.

The use of face-to-face interviews with borderline patients helps the therapist to be aware of the patient's nonverbal behavior. This is often an important clue to his or her character defenses, and also assists the therapist in focusing on the patient's here-and-now reality. Unlike some clinicians, Kernberg does not think that frequent sessions stimulate too much regression if the treatment is conducted so that the patient's excessive needs are not gratified and acting-out is prevented. In fact, he regards once a week treatment as problematic in that it usually results in a therapist's excessive preoccupation with the patient's life between sessions. This makes the use of an interpretative approach more difficult.

A firm treatment structure is necessary because borderline patients have difficulties with time and consistency and tend to deviate from established routines. It is important to focus initially on the patient's current behavior and relationships as fully as possible, since these are more reliable sources of data about the patient's characteristic difficulties than his or her recounting and interpretation of past events. It is essential to evaluate the need for the kinds of supports equivalent to those found in more structured settings, such as hospitals or residential treatment settings, in order to contain the patient's tendency to act-out impulsively and destructively. These may include day hospitals, work, school, and leisure-time activities and routines, auxiliary treatment modalities, self-help groups such as AA and NA, and clear expectations and rules. Sometimes structure can be provided through the use of an auxiliary therapist such as a social worker, who functions in a supportive and reality-oriented way with the patient, and thereby frees the primary therapist to engage in more modifying treatments. This approach is inevitably accompanied by the patient's splitting of the therapists into the "good" one and the "bad" one, but since the auxiliary and primary therapists communicate with one another, such splitting can be diagnosed and utilized in the patient's treatment.

The therapist needs to play an active role in setting limits on the destructive expression of aggression or other impulses in the session and on other forms of acting-out or requests for special treatment. For example, the therapist may ask a patient to refrain from yelling or refuse to answer personal questions. Establishing a clear verbal or written contract about the patient's responsibilities in controlling his or her potentially destructive behavior, as well as the consequences of being unable to do so is important in many instances (Kernberg et al., 1989). For example, with a patient who smokes marijuana before coming to sessions, the therapist will tell him or her that he or she will not be talked to under the influence; with a patient who drinks excessively on weekends when lonely, the therapist will indicate that the patient must develop other means of soothing herself and stick to them or the treatment will be terminated until such time as the drinking is under control; with a patient who calls the therapist frequently at night when he becomes panicky, the therapist will convey that the patient should not call, that the therapist will hang up if the patient telephones, and that the patient should go to an emergency room if he or she gets too desperate; and with a patient who repeatedly threatens suicide, the therapist might say that if the patient cannot control his or her suicidal behavior, the patient will be hospitalized and the therapist will not treat the patient until he or she is discharged. In setting contracts of this kind, Kernberg suggests that the therapist start with less restrictive limits and consequences and use more restrictive ones only if necessary. In many instances, it will be important to interpret the patient's resistance to agreeing to or following the contract. The therapist, however, should continue to insist on rather than delay the establishment of limits even if this means ending the treatment if the patient is unwilling or unable to cooperate in this way.

Sometimes patients are so chronically suicidal or otherwise destructive that any treatment that attempts to modify their core pathology activates their acting-out. In these instances it is preferable to provide long-term in-patient treatment (see Chapter 9) that combines an expressive approach with protection and structure, than to attempt an out-patient supportive psychotherapy that does not reach the roots of their difficulties. Although the risk of severe acting-out and suicide may always be present, some of these cases can be treated on an out-patient basis, especially when patients can be trusted to communicate their thoughts and feelings openly and to adhere to the established ground rules (Kernberg, 1984). Even with these patients, however, brief hospitalizations may be necessary at times.

While Kernberg generally is opposed to using minor or major tranquilizers with borderline patients, he does utilize antidepressants in those patients who manifest a true affective disorder alongside of their personality difficulties. Since borderline patients typically present with complaints of depression, a careful evaluation should be made of whether or not they have a "true" affective disorder.

Because borderline individuals' characteristic defenses of denial, splitting, and projective identification lead to distortions of their interpersonal relationships and often glaring omissions of important details of their behavior, contact between the therapist and other professionals and significant others may need to be built into their treatment. Only in this way can the therapist gain a full picture of the significant aspects of a patient's life that may otherwise be kept out of the sessions. Such contact may also help to lessen the negative consequences of the patient's primitive defenses that often result in the "splitting" of those in his or her life into all "good" or all "bad." Family members, friends, and helpers may begin to view one another in terms of these one-dimensional stereotypes, blame or become competitive with one another, and even unwittingly sabotage therapeutic efforts. Issues of confidentiality and expectations regarding the nature of such contact with a patient's significant others should be worked out carefully and early in the treatment. The prevention, diagnosis, and resolution of the collaborative difficulties that may be activated by a patient's splitting of those professionals who are trying to help into "good" and "bad," will also need to be addressed.

The Nature of the Therapeutic Relationship

Therapeutic Neutrality

An indispensable feature of Kernberg's treatment model is the therapist's adherence to a technically neutral position or attitude in his or her interventions. Technical neutrality requires that the therapist maintains an equal distance from the patient's id, ego, and superego instead of siding with or against one of these mental structures as might be characteristic of supportive psychotherapy or treatments that combine supportive and expressive techniques. Likewise, the therapist must remain "abstinent" in the sense of refraining from giving in to the patient's demands for transference gratification. Instead, such requests or expectations should be explored and interpreted. For example, a technically neutral response to a patient who arrives at a session and enthusiastically tells the therapist of a promotion and waits expectantly for some positive reaction would be: "Let us try to understand why it is so important that I tell you I am pleased with your success." Or, to another patient who describes his or her tendency to break off close relationships when frustrated only to feel very depressed afterward, the therapist might say: "It seems important to consider why you continue to act in ways that seem to lead you to feel badly." A violation of technical neutrality in the first example would be reflected in the therapist gratifying the patient's need for a demonstrable sign of the therapist's pleasure. In the second example a non-neutral therapist might have encouraged the patient to think about the consequences of impulsively terminating a relationship before doing so in order to prevent feeling regretful later.

Detours from technical neutrality compromise the therapist's ability to confront and interpret the patient's pathological defenses and behavior. They should therefore be avoided. While the acting-out potential of some patients will induce the therapist to abandon such neutrality at times, it is preferable to structure the patient's life outside of the sessions and to set clear limits on the patient's behavior so that these disruptions are minimized.

In his response to those who have equated technical neutrality with a lack of humanness and empathy Kernberg (1984) has indicated that caring, personal warmth, and respect are important therapeutic qualities. Likewise, the therapist must provide a "holding" or "containing" function in which the therapist absorbs and organizes the patient's chaotic inner experience, withstands the patient's aggression without retaliation, and maintains an attitude of concern and emotional availability. He goes on to say, however, that true empathy with patients who are quite contradictory and who split off crucial feeling states requires the therapist to be in tune emotionally not only with the patient's subjective experience or with what is being communicated at a given moment, but also with what is being split off. As the therapist attempts to integrate the split off parts, the patient may become more uncomfortable and defensive. It may look as if the therapist is attacking the patient because of the therapist's efforts to help the patient accept parts of himself or herself that the patient resists acknowledging.

The Therapeutic Alliance and the Transference

The term therapeutic alliance, sometimes called the working or helping alliance, describes the relationship between the patient's and therapist's rational egos, which come together around the helping task and arrangements (Greenson, 1967). It is commonly believed that the formation of this partnership is one of the first steps in any psychotherapy. Higher functioning patients typically possess an observing ego that enables them to weather the host of stormy transference reactions that develop inevitably during treatment. They remain aware at some level, for example, that despite experiencing the therapist as a punitive father figure he is, in reality, someone who is trying to be helpful. While the intensity of some transference reactions may interfere with accurate perceptions at times, the therapist generally is able to strengthen the alliance by appealing to the patient's understanding of the therapeutic task and the nature of the treatment process, or by reminding the patient of the more positive aspects of the relationship. Likewise, patients who show reasonably good ego functioning tend to display transferences that are fairly consistent over time and about which they show some awareness themselves. Moreover, since their defenses center on repression and other higher level mechanisms, they do not split off contradictory reactions that may surface suddenly in disruptive ways. Nor do their defenses typically distort their perceptions dramatically.

With psychotic patients the capacity to form and maintain a therapeutic alliance may be grossly hampered by problems in reality testing and loss of ego boundaries. Psychotic transference reactions develop in which patients do not experience the therapist as a separate person at any level. With borderline patients, however, the therapeutic alliance is tenuous for somewhat different reasons. While maintaining the capacity for reality testing generally, these individuals form intense, primitive reactions even very early in treatment that temporarily overwhelm the observing ego. Since early self- and object-representations have not been integrated, the borderline patient's transference reactions often are initially chaotic and changing. Sometimes a powerful transference occurs in the patient's first telephone contact or meeting with a therapist.

Since splitting and the related mechanisms of denial, idealization, devaluation, omnipotent control, and projective identification ward off the patient's aggression, what may appear overtly as a positive transference reaction may hide a more covert set of feelings that are equally important to understand. Intense anger that is denied and projected onto the therapist may lead to impulsive acting-out or destruction of the therapeutic relationship.

These special features require a different focus in the work with borderline patients. The main question therapeutically is how to deal with the aggressive impulses and resultant defenses that make it repeatedly difficult for these patients to develop and maintain a stable working relationship. This requires an active approach from the beginning of treatment, when the therapist must identify the patient's confusing and often latent negative transference reactions and primitive defenses that distort or threaten the treatment. It is potentially disastrous to sit back and allow what appears to be an intense positive feeling — for example, idealization — to develop, since the presence of splitting may be masking more negative and potentially destructive reactions. Likewise, it is not useful in the long run to attempt to build the positive alliance through supportive means since this leads to further splitting off and possible acting out of aggression.

The Therapist as an Objective Expert

A controversial assumption underlying the emphasis on technical neutrality is that the therapist is able to objectively observe the patient's pathology in the treatment situation if the therapist manages his or her behavior so that it does not impinge on the patient. If the therapist is able to maintain a technically neutral position, then whatever the patient presents reflects his or her own personality rather than the influence of the therapist. Because borderline patients' defenses lead to a distortion of their perceptions of themselves and others, the therapist's view of reality is seen as more accurate and reliable. Thus, the therapist is more of an expert on what patients are experiencing than they are themselves. The therapist's role is to . . . "confront the patient's distortions, demonstrate their inappropriateness, clarify the underlying aggressive infiltrates and the defensive projections and splits, restore and strengthen the capacity of the patient's ego to perceive reality correctly" (Lang, 1987, p. 144).

Main Techniques and Principal Features

The maintenance of technical neutrality whenever possible is in keeping with an emphasis on the use of techniques such as clarification, confrontation, and interpretation rather than reassurance, suggestion, encouragement, and manipulation as major tools in the treatment of borderline patients. The interpretative function of the therapist takes precedence over the experiential aspects of the treatment process in promoting structural change. This stress on content rather than process is a distinctive feature of this model (Waldinger & Gunderson, 1987). Since borderline personality structure is impervious to, often prevents the development of, or actively destroys positive relationship experiences, new types of relating are the outcome of treatment rather than a means for achieving therapeutic success. Further, the ways in which patients distort or attempt to destroy meaningful relationships must be addressed systematically.

The therapist's provision of a respectful and caring human relationship and a "holding" or "containing" environment over the course of the treatment does contribute to the patient's improvement, particularly with those who have been exposed to extreme abuse or neglect. For them the therapist's attention and concern are better than anything they have previously experienced. Kernberg explicitly cautions, however, against the therapist's deliberate use of the relationship to repair patients' early developmental trauma. He argues that "what really strengthens the patient's ego is not the gratification of needs in the here-and-now that were denied in the there-and-then but a coming to terms with past frustrations and limitations . . . (Kernberg, 1984, p. 121).

Within the general framework for the treatment discussed above the technically neutral therapist uses four main techniques in the expressive psychotherapy of borderline patients—clarification, confrontation, interpretation, and transference interpretation. Sometimes the therapist may rely on one of these techniques more than others. On other occasions they may be used sequentially.

Clarification

Clarification implies a nonchallenging, cognitive exploration of what the patient is communicating so that the therapist is able to understand the patient more fully. It focuses on what is incomplete, vague, discrepant, or contradictory and can be used to test the limits of the patient's awareness and conscious understanding of the implications of what is being said. The following example shows the therapist's efforts to understand the patient's fluctuating plans for her immediate future and whether the patient herself was able to acknowledge how seemingly contradictory she was being.

AMELIA: I had a great weekend. I went to visit my friend, Barbara, in Pennsylvania. She lives in a real artists' community and I decided that that's where I want to be. I'm ready to move but I don't know whether to sublet or keep my apartment in New York.

THERAPIST: I was under the impression from our conversation on Friday that you had made a firm decision to stay in the city and go on for further training. What has happened in the meantime to change your mind?

AMELIA: I mailed in the applications to school last week. By the way, my mother called and said she would lend me the money for tuition. Can you imagine? That bitch! I never know what she's going to do next.

THERAPIST: Are you thinking about taking her up on her offer?

AMELIA: No! I told you that I'm moving to Pennsylvania! Can't you understand English?

THERAPIST: You seem angry with me for trying to understand what you want to do. Can you tell me why?

AMELIA: I'm not angry! I just wish you'd pay attention to what I'm saying. There was something else I wanted to tell you. I got a letter from Jack in Arizona. He said I could borrow his car if I moved out there and that the social scene for women is really great with all the single men around. I think I may go for a visit to check it out.

THERAPIST: You seem to have many different plans. What are your feelings about that?

Confrontation

Clarification lays the groundwork for confrontation and interpretation. Confrontation involves the therapist's efforts to foster the patient's awareness of, and to help the patient bring together, contradictory aspects of his or her thoughts, feelings, and behavior. The therapist does this by presenting the patient with what the therapist observes to be confusing or discrepant in what the patient is saying (at the moment or over time) in order to see if the patient can acknowledge the seeming contradictions. The therapist then asks the patient to explain or reflect on the meaning of these discrepancies, and may also draw attention to the connection between "here-and-now" interactions and similar problems in other areas of the patient's life (Kernberg, 1977). Since the borderline patient generally is actively trying not to acknowledge intolerable feeling states or unfavorable characteristics, he or she will likely experience even tactful or gentle confrontations as unempathic or even as assaults. These often activate defensive or angry reactions, as is shown below. Some patients, however, become more realistic in the face of confrontation.

THERAPIST: I'm somewhat puzzled about what you want to do?

AMELIA: I'm not confused. I know exactly what I want.

THERAPIST: Can you appreciate why I'm somewhat puzzled on the basis of what you're telling me?

AMELIA: No.

THERAPIST: Well, how do you understand the fact that you seem to have three totally different plans and present each one as if it's the only one while at the same time you still hold on to the others that you claim to have discarded.

AMELIA: What do you mean?

THERAPIST: Two weeks ago you were moving to Arizona in order to increase your chances of getting married. Last week you were staying in New York and continuing in school and didn't want to talk about Arizona. Today you announced that you were going to move to Pennsylvania imminently but then seemed interested in your mother's decision to lend you tuition and Jack's offer of his car and news about Arizona's social scene.

AMELIA: So what?

THERAPIST: You seem angry about my raising this with you.

AMELIA: What is your problem? Why do you have to be such a wet blanket?

THERAPIST: Can we talk about why it is so difficult for you when I try to understand the reasoning behind your conflicting plans? The reason you came into treatment was that you felt you couldn't get your life together. When I try to help you to think things through, you get angry with me.

AMELIA: I feel like you're questioning my every feeling.

Interpretation

Interpretation goes beyond helping the patient to explore and explain his or her contradictory or problematic thoughts, feelings, and behavior. It involves presenting patients with possible explanations of the underlying motives for their defenses, transference reactions, or other self-destructive and self-defeating behavior. Such interpretations have an ego strengthening effect on borderline patients. The therapist usually interprets dominant themes in the sessions, works from surface to depth in the sense that material closer to consciousness is interpreted before unconscious material, addresses the patient's lack of awareness of significant feelings, and comments on the conflictual aspects of the patient's thoughts, feelings, and behavior. However, not all interpretations are complete in the sense that they link present behavior to the past. Particularly in the early phases of the treatment of borderline patients interpretations should focus on the "here-and-now" meaning of behavior, as the following example shows, since patients' memories of their childhood past are too filled with distortions for firm connections to be made between present and past. They should always begin with the establishment of a common reality about what has occurred (Kernberg, 1989).

Amelia: You have this agenda for me to think about everything I do before I do it. You're such a bore!

THERAPIST: Can you tell me why it makes you so angry when I question you?

AMELIA: So I'm angry. Just leave me alone!

THERAPIST: Perhaps the reason that it's so difficult for you to even consider weighing the pros and cons of your various options is that you always have to feel totally right and certain, as if having any doubts or questions means that you are weak and vulnerable? It's more important for you to come across to yourself and others as decisive and in control even if you choose the wrong course of action than to appear not to know what you want.

AMELIA: I can't stand indecision. I know what I want. No one is going to tell me what to do.

THERAPIST: Perhaps it is your one need for control that makes you convinced that I am trying to tell you what to do when I am merely trying to understand you?

AMELIA: You're really an expert at twisting things.

THERAPIST: Why would I do that?

Transference Interpretation

The therapist uses clarification, confrontation, and interpretation to make the patient aware of the nature of his or her reactions to the therapist that are based on the patient's primitive defenses. A full transference interpretation links these responses to their origins in the patient's past perceptions of others.

> THERAPIST: Perhaps when I question you about your contradictory plans you think I'm treating you the way you experienced your father, who made you feel weak and stupid? Now with me it's very important that you feel you are in total control.
>
> AMELIA: So what?
>
> THERAPIST: If I go along with your ever changing plans, never question you, and refrain from helping you think through what you really want to do, then I'm not helping you, but if I do question you, you experience me as trying to control, blame, and humiliate you the way you felt your father did. You become enraged and have to attack me. I think you show this rage in other situations too when anyone questions you.

Confrontation and Interpretation of the Defenses that Threaten the Therapeutic Alliance

Systematic attention to the transference and to the patient's primitive defenses is the cornerstone of an expressive approach even in the earliest stages. The therapist should confront and interpret the latent negative transference reactions and primitive defenses since these interventions will strengthen the therapeutic alliance and improve the patient's observing ego in the short-run.

The interpretive process should initially be confined to the patient's current interactions with the therapist rather than include linkages to the patient's past relationships with parental figures or significant others. Borderline patients have difficulties differentiating transference objects from real past objects, and their childhood memories are filled with distortions. Thus, the therapist's efforts to connect present to past will be based on erroneous information and conclusions about the nature of the patient's past experiences. In the vignette below the therapist confronts and interprets the patient's defensive idealization of him because of the past history of the patient's abrupt and premature terminations from several other therapists whom he also had initially admired. The therapist does not link her interpretation of the patient's behavior to his childhood past.

> RON: I was telling a friend of mine that you are the most sensitive therapist I've ever had. You make the others look like total incompetents by comparison.
>
> THERAPIST: Tell me more about that.

RON: They were all idiots. I don't know how I could have thought they were so great at first. They even had the nerve to keep trying to get me to pay for the sessions that *they* loused up!

THERAPIST: What went wrong?

RON: They were incompetent.

THERAPIST: Can you say a little more about the radical change in your feelings about them?

RON: They were okay for awhile and then they turned out to be frauds. They all made pronouncements as if they knew it all, and then they turned out to be not so perfect themselves. Can you imagine a shrink driving a cheap car or wearing *white* socks or making a mistake in billing?

THERAPIST: But how do you understand the fact that you admired them for what seemed to be their sensitivity and skill one minute, and then viewed them as the scum of the earth the next, just because their personal tastes seemed to differ from yours?

RON: I don't know why you're pursuing this! What's your point?

THERAPIST: Now you're getting angry at me when a minute ago you thought I was the greatest.

RON: A minute ago you weren't giving me a hard time.

THERAPIST: I am just puzzled. You tell me how much you admire me, but if I ask you to explain some of your contradictory and shifting feelings, you turn on me as you did your other therapists. Perhaps you need to see me as perfect in order to protect me from your envy and hatred of my position?

RON: You are acting like God.

THERAPIST: I think you have quite a lot of anger at and fear of me. If you don't appease me by telling me that you admire me, who knows what I will do?

RON: So I have a lot of anger. So what?

THERAPIST: You will turn your rage on me eventually and view me as you did the other therapists. You might even leave treatment again feeling justified in getting away from my incompetence.

Connecting the Patient's Transference Reactions and Defenses to Other Current Situations

Once the therapist understands the nature of the patient's main transferences and the ways in which primitive defenses distort the treatment relationship, it is important for the therapist to link the patient's feelings and behavior in the treatment to his or her current difficulties with others. The therapist again should refrain initially from explaining the patient's problems with others in terms of the repetition of past relationships. Instead, the therapist should focus on how the patient distorts his or her interactions with and perceptions of others, as the next example shows. This will diminish the patient's defensiveness and improve reality testing temporarily.

RON: My boss is a real asshole. He's constantly looking over my shoulder. Doesn't he think I have any intelligence? He's such a bureaucrat. I thought he would be different at first. He seemed like a good guy. Now I can't stand him. I'm sure he's going to fire me if I don't leave first. I just can't get myself to be nice to him.

THERAPIST: Do you think it's possible that you're doing the same thing with him that you've done so many times before?

RON: I can't help it if I keep running into real incompetents who have to show how important and smart they are at my expense. Do you think I'm supposed to always take what's dished out?

THERAPIST: Doesn't it seem possible that it is you who can't stand being subservient to your boss, and that you try to cover up your hatred of his position by seeming to look up to him? Then you get angry and demean him when he exercises his authority just as you have done with other bosses, therapists, and even with me.

RON: How do I do that with you?

THERAPIST: You tell me that I am the most sensitive therapist you have ever known and then you become annoyed and sarcastic when I make a comment that displeases you.

RON: Is that a crime?

THERAPIST: Do you think that's what I'm saying?

RON: I guess not. Maybe I do have a chip on my shoulder at times.

Allowing the Less Primitive Positive Transference to Develop

While Kernberg warns the therapists of borderline patients not to be misled by many seemingly positive transference developments that may actually reflect a defensive idealization, he indicates that there are "non-specific" positive features of all good therapeutic encounters that foster the treatment and which do not need to be explored. It is important to accept rather than to confront the patient's less charged positive feelings in order to foster the therapeutic alliance. It would be ill-advised for the therapist to comment on signs or expressions of the patient's positive feelings about treatment when these seem appropriate rather than extreme or defensive reactions, as in the following vignette. Sometimes it may be difficult, however, for the therapist to differentiate between these two types of responses.

JEFF: I've been feeling a little better lately.

THERAPIST: Tell me a little more about that.

JEFF: I feel less angry and I seem to be handling things better. I look forward to our sessions. I just wanted to let you know.

THERAPIST: It seems important that you share that with me.

JEFF: I dump so much garbage in here. I wanted to let you know the good things too. I usually find it easier to complain.

THERAPIST: You said you were handling things better. Can you give me an example?

JEFF: I feel surer of myself when I have to approach the judge at a trial. Yesterday Judge Black made a sarcastic remark when I asked for another postponement for my client. I kept my cool and he granted it. I didn't get so angry.

Confrontation and Interpretation of the Patient's Distortions of the Therapist's Interventions

The therapist's efforts to confront and interpret the patient's latent or manifest negative transference reactions and primitive defenses are not automatically accepted by the patient. Since the therapist's interventions are intended to obstruct the very defenses that borderline patients use to protect themselves, resistance is inevitable. This usually takes the form of continuing, if not escalating, distortions of the therapist's motivations, and attacks on his or her character or competence. The appropriate intervention in these instances is to interpret the patient's reactions as further evidence of primitive defenses, as is exemplified below, rather than to back down or to soothe the patient in the face of his or her intense, intimidating, and provocative responses. This tactic eventually helps to diminish the patient's extreme reactions.

TINA: I'm quitting treatment. Send me a bill. That's all you care about anyway!

THERAPIST: Can you tell me what's making you so angry that you want to leave treatment?

TINA: You're not going to talk me out of leaving you. All you want to do is exploit me and your fees are too high anyway. You don't really care about me. You enjoy making money as a result of other peoples' suffering.

THERAPIST: I'm really puzzled by your reaction because on Friday you told me how I am the only one who is really there for you and how you trust me completely.

TINA: That was Friday! Today is Monday and I don't trust you anymore.

THERAPIST: Perhaps when I'm not available to you on the weekend you become enraged that I have a life apart from you? You then think that I am angry with you and trying to take advantage of you.

TINA: You're not going to manipulate me into staying. I know your game!

THERAPIST: Why would I be trying to manipulate you?

TINA: What did you say? Can you repeat what you said? You are not enunciating clearly.

THERAPIST: I guess you can't even listen to what I'm saying because it gives me too much power over you and you want to have control over me. You have to wipe me out or disagree with me, without even thinking about what I'm saying, in order to make sure that I know you're the boss.

TINA: I don't know why you can't see me on Saturdays. That's when I need you. What good are you?

THERAPIST: Isn't it a little contradictory to feel that I should see you on Saturdays on the one hand and to be quitting treatment on the other? What's going on?

TINA: You're too smart for me. You understand me too well. I'm just trying to pick a fight with you. So my parents and I had a fight Saturday and I got really upset.

Integration of Self- and Object-Representations

There are three sometimes overlapping steps to helping patients to integrate their split off internalized images of themselves and others. In the first step the therapist attempts to understand and engage the patient in reflecting on the contradictory part self- and object-representations that emerge at different times. The therapist asks himself or herself how the patient is coming across now in comparison to other times, and asks the patient to explain the differences in the way he or she portrays himself or herself or others? Secondly, the therapist focuses on the self- and object-representations and their interactions that are expressed in the transference and attempts to evaluate "Who is doing what to whom?" or "Who is experiencing what from whom?" (Kernberg, 1984, p. 107). In the third step the therapist helps the patient to connect his or her part-object relations transferences and what they represent to one another. This process, which is illustrated below, goes on repetitively and it can take a long time before any lasting integration occurs. It is a difficult process because the very defenses that the therapist confronts serve to prevent such integration, and the patient frequently responds to the therapist's interventions with increasing defensiveness. These reactions, in turn, need to be addressed.

In the case of Nancy, a 23-year-old young woman, the therapist was unable to understand her initial communications because Nancy tended to jump from topic to topic and described a confusing picture of herself and others. Soon, however, the therapist was able to discern several distinct patterns. At times Nancy presented herself as a victim of others' lack of appreciation, insensitivity, and exploitation. On these occasions she portrayed herself as a helpless child who was being treated unfairly by powerful and abusive caretakers—for example, her parents, boss, intimate friends, and the therapist. A second pattern revealed itself when she would feel insecure and inadequate, and idealize those around her to whom she looked for advice, approval, and validation and whom she protected from criticism. A third pattern was reflected in Nancy's experience of herself as powerful and self-righteous. She then felt justified in verbally attacking those around her for their weakness and failures.

Nancy sometimes actually seemed to have insight into her problems, but this understanding did not seem to carry over into her behavior outside treatment and she quickly escalated in her more extreme reactions. With this understanding of Nancy's fluctuating self- and object-representations the therapist identified each facet of Nancy when it was presented and asked Nancy to consider and explain the other facets that she had previously expressed, both in discussing her life and in the transference itself.

NANCY: My mother would not give me the telephone number of where she and my father are staying on vacation. It's bad enough that they're going away on the weekend before my birthday. She doesn't care about me and whether I'm alone. I could get sick and die and she wouldn't care. She's such a bitch and my father lets her get away with it. He has no backbone.

THERAPIST: Today you are portraying yourself as a child without any resources who needs her parents to take care of her, and you are describing your parents as totally insensitive, selfish, and uncaring.

NANCY: They are totally selfish and they don't care! I can't stand them!

THERAPIST: Just last week you told me how much you loved them and how fearful you were that they would die. You became enraged at me and defended them when I pointed out that you felt they were rarely there for you. How do you understand the change in your feelings?

NANCY: They change.

THERAPIST: But you describe them in such totally opposite ways. Either they're all "good" or all "bad."

NANCY: I screamed at my mother. I told her that if she didn't give me the telephone number she might find me dead when she came home. She got hysterical and accused me of being a tyrant.

THERAPIST: It's quite a contradiction, don't you think?. You get desperate and feel she's abandoning you but then you turn the tables on her. You become the all-powerful one and she feels like your victim.

NANCY: Do I have to listen to this? What are you trying to do? I don't pay you to attack me. You don't care about me. I bet you can't wait until the session is over. You're probably thinking about how you're going to spend my fee while you're talking to me.

THERAPIST: Right now you are experiencing yourself in relation to me the way you feel with your mother. You are the victim and I am the abuser and you have the right to attack me for abusing you. Just a little while ago you saw me as someone who cared about you and who could help you. Aren't I still the same person?

NANCY: No. You changed.

THERAPIST: I think the changes go on in you. You become easily enraged when you feel you can't control the people around you. You can't accept your need to control others and your intense anger. Instead you see everyone else as trying to hurt you and you provoke them until they do. Then you feel justified in your perceptions of their maltreatment of you and let your temper loose.

NANCY: I don't feel powerful. I feel inadequate. I need people to take care of me.

THERAPIST: It is easier for you to feel that way at times then to accept your need to control others and your anger. You seem to idealize others and treat them as if they're strong and you're weak.

NANCY: You really love to talk. You should have been a lawyer.

THERAPIST: I guess ridiculing me is your way of dismissing what I have to say so that you don't have to look at the different sides of yourself.

Working with Higher Level Defenses and Transferences

When the borderline individual's part self- and object-representations begin to coalesce and the more destructive aspects of their behavior are modulated, the therapist can focus on helping the patient to overcome the splitting that dominates his or her inner life. This is done through systematic interpretation of the conflicts that are active within the patient. As the patient becomes more aware of ambivalent feelings, more expressive of his or her subjective experience, more able to describe others realistically, and more truly self-reflective, the therapist can address the patient's higher level defenses, transference reactions, and intersystemic (id, ego, superego) conflicts. In this phase genetic interpretations that link current behavior to past experiences can be made since the patient is able to be more accurate in communicating about the past.

Countertransference Issues

While the classical view of countertransference refers to the therapist's emotional reactions to the patient that are based on the therapist's own unresolved unconscious conflicts, the totalistic conception, to which Kernberg subscribes, defines countertransference more broadly. This view includes all of the therapist's *conscious* and *unconscious* reactions to the patient, including those that are *induced* by the patient's personality, psychopathology, and life situation. It encompasses what Winnicott (1949) termed "objective countertransference" in referring to the natural or quite justifiable reactions of the therapist to extreme aspects of the patient's behavior, what Racker (1957) called "concordant identification," in which the therapist experiences the main emotion that the patient is feeling at a given time, and "complementary identification," in which the therapist experiences the feeling that the patient has put into him or her as a transference object at the same time that the patient experiences an emotion in relationship to that perceived transference object. For example, in concordant identification the therapist's empathic immersion in the patient's experience may lead him or her to experience the patient's rage. This is a common experience as a result of the borderline patient's frequent use of projective identification in which he or she continues to have an impulse, generally an angry one, which at the same time is projected onto the therapist who then is feared as an enemy who must be controlled. While patients utilize this mechanism in order to rid themselves of unacceptable hostility, they still experience their own anger but feel it is a justifiable reaction to the therapist who has become the target of their projections. In complementary identification the therapist may begin to feel like a harsh and controlling figure while the patient experiences a fear of the therapist that is related to his or her perception of the therapist as an enemy.

While those who rely on the classical definition of countertransference emphasize its potentially disruptive influence on the treatment, those who use the totalistic conception regard countertransference reactions as potentially diagnostic of what is really occurring in the patient's inner life. The main treatment implications of this latter view involve the therapist's ability to use his or her countertransference reactions to understand the nature of the patient's internalized object relations as they appear in the transference. This shifts the focus from the therapist's assumption of full responsibility for his or her reactions to the patient to his or her attending to what in the patient or in the patient's perceived relationship to others is being recreated in the transference and countertransference.

In the example above the therapist became aware of her rising anger at Nancy and of a wish to tell Nancy to get out of her office when Nancy was ridiculing her for thinking about her fee during the session. She quickly realized that she was being provoked to act in an abusive and rejecting manner by Nancy, who was perceiving herself as a weak and helpless victim of the therapist's power in order to ward off her wish to control the therapist (mother) and her rage at not being able to do so. With this awareness the therapist became calm internally and interpreted the object relation and projective identification that was being enacted in the treatment.

While focusing on the problem of induced countertransference, Kernberg clearly acknowledges that there is a danger that the therapist's reactions will obstruct the treatment if they are not understood and resolved. Because of the intense, often primitive, and unrelenting nature of borderline patients' responses—particularly aggression, along with projective identification—therapists are at risk to counterattack, submit to, withdraw from, or omnipotently dedicate themselves to the treatment of the patient as their own early identifications and defenses are stirred up. Sometimes chronic countertransference reactions lead to therapeutic stalemates. In order to withstand the patient's assaults, therapists should be alert to the patient's destructive impulses, and of the possibility of these being mobilized in themselves, and remain committed to helping the patient despite the patient's "badness."

KERNBERG'S SUPPORTIVE PSYCHOTHERAPY

Generally, traditional forms of supportive psychotherapy aim at restoring, maintaining, or enhancing an individual's adaptive functioning without attempting to modify or change basic and entrenched personality traits, defenses, and structure or to resolve unconscious conflicts. The therapist focuses on the patient's current reality rather than on past behavior and fantasies, and attempts to minimize regression and to strengthen defenses. The real relationship between therapist and patient or the benign positive transference, rather than any intense positive and negative transference reactions, is encouraged. Sometimes the therapist attempts to provide a "corrective emotional experience" and to build ego where there are deficits. Sessions usually occur less frequently than is true of expressive psychotherapy. Techniques such as ventilation, reassurance, rational discussion, education, advice, and environmental manipulation are preferred over more reflective and interpretive ones (Goldstein, 1984; Kernberg, 1984; Knight, 1953b; and Zetzel, 1971).

On the basis of the findings of the Psychotherapy Research Project of the Menninger Foundation (Kernberg et al., 1972), Kernberg concluded that while supportive psychotherapy might lead to some improvement in a patient's subjective state and behavior in the short-run, it tended to perpetuate pathological defenses, poor ego functioning, and identity disturbances in the long-run. Remaining vulnerable, borderline patients who received such treatment might become "lifers," requiring the interminable presence of a therapist in order to maintain their functioning. Emphasizing the use of expressive psychotherapy with borderline patients, Kernberg did not offer an alternative approach until recently when he described a unique variant of supportive treatment. He still clearly regards this type of treatment as a "last resort — when other modes must be ruled out" (Kernberg, 1984, p. 151).

Treatment Goals and Framework

The main goal of Kernberg's supportive psychotherapy is to help patients to function more adaptively. More specific objectives are individualized and range from modest attempts at helping patients to gain control over destructive behavior, to be more autonomous within their limitations, and sometimes to achieve greater independent living without chronically relying on protective environmental structures such as day hospitals. Kernberg advocates a systematic, though non-interpretive attempt at helping patients to identify and understand the presence and disorganizing effects of primitive defenses, negative transference reactions, and characteristic problems in their interpersonal relationships and social functioning.

A clear and consistent structure should be established in supportive psychotherapy so that the patient's efforts to deviate from this framework can be recognized and understood. While the frequency of sessions varies, the decision about this should rest on an evaluation of the patient's needs and characteristics. It may be useful for some patients to see the therapist more often during a life crisis or if they have difficulty maintaining a sense of connection. The less frequently that the patient is seen, the harder it may be for the therapist to track what is most relevant to work on in the treatment. Generally, it will be necessary for the therapist to actively seek out information about the patient's life between sessions, to work at making connections from one session to another, and to establish a sufficient degree of external structure, along with a clear understanding about the nature of the therapist's and patient's mutual responsibilities for the treatment.

The Nature of the Therapeutic Relationship

In supportive treatment the therapist actively helps the patient to understand and deal with the demands of external reality, and also fosters the appropriate expression of the patient's emotional needs. Thus, the therapist does not remain neutral with respect to his or her interventions. At the same time, the therapist does not encourage the activation of the patient's primitive transferences, dependency, or magical expectations by relying unnecessarily on too much direct advice, reassurance, or involvement in the patient's life. While some of these interventions may be necessary, every effort should be made to convey to the patient that the therapist has respect for the patient's capacities to think and do for himself or herself. Likewise, the therapist does not attempt to provide the patient with an emotionally corrective relationship experience that aims to repair earlier deficits. While the therapist's concern for the patient over time may have positive effects, the therapist focuses on helping the patient both to understand the impact of his or her feelings and behaviors and to modulate these in accord with reality. One can characterize the therapist's role as that of a teacher about the nature of reality and appropriate behavior.

Main Techniques and Principal Features

A Focus on Primitive Defenses

The main tool in supportive psychotherapy with borderline patients involves the identification of the primitive defenses that the patient uses and their problematic effects. In a supportive approach the therapist *does not* interpret these defenses as would be the case in expressive psychotherapy but instead points them out and educates the patient to recognize their presence and impact on current interpersonal relationships and social functioning. Thus, the therapist must consistently though tactfully challenge the patient when he or she presents distortions of reality and maladaptive responses as shown below.

NANCY: I'm sick and tired of Emily keeping me waiting. She was ½ hour late yesterday for dinner. I'm going to break-off my relationship with her. I don't like her any more.

THERAPIST: Does she always keep you waiting or are you just mad because you had to wait for her yesterday?

NANCY: I don't know who she thinks I am. I'm not her slave.

THERAPIST: Did she give you a reason for being late?

NANCY: She said her boss needed her to type something.

THERAPIST: Don't you believe her?

NANCY: I just don't like her any more.

THERAPIST: You often tend to end relationships when you feel frustrated or put down in some way, even if the person doesn't intend to hurt you. When you are angry you forget a person's good traits and your positive feelings for them. Later you miss them.

NANCY: Are you saying that I shouldn't break up with Emily?

THERAPIST: I think that when you find yourself not liking someone any more and wanting to end the relationship suddenly, it is important to realize that this is what you do when you get frustrated and that later you generally regret your actions.

NANCY: So what should I do instead?

THERAPIST: Perhaps it would be better to wait a while and try to remember what you liked about Emily, and whether you really think she always is trying to hurt you? Is she as "bad" as you think at the moment?

NANCY: I don't want to wait.

THERAPIST: Of course what you do is up to you, but I can only say that when you act on your angry feelings you often defeat yourself.

Work with the Negative Transference

While supportive psychotherapy reduces the intensity of the patient's transference reactions generally, it does not do so completely. The therapist who hopes to build a positive transference in order to further the treatment and to strengthen the patient's ego through the process of identification by avoiding dealing with negative reactions will make a serious error. Borderline patients are not generally capable of forming and maintaining such positive attachments without concurrent negative reactions and distortions of their relationships as a result of their primitive defenses. A second and related technical intervention in supportive psychotherapy is the therapist's pointing out of the patient's latent and negative transference reactions, and their possible connection to the patient's characteristic ways of relating to others.

NANCY: I've been feeling very positive toward you lately. You really are there for me. I look forward to seeing you. I don't feel so alone.

THERAPIST: While you feel that way today, last week you were ready to leave treatment because I seemed cold and indifferent.

NANCY: Why do you always bring up my anger?

THERAPIST: I'm a little concerned that despite your positive feelings, your anger will lead you to quit treatment suddenly just as you do with friendships.

NANCY: But I love you.

THERAPIST: Sometimes you have two sets of feelings. You feel positive when you're with a person and then you feel quite angry when they're not there to meet your needs, like with Emily. You have quick changes of heart. You feel good one minute and then you get hurt and angry and want to toss her away.

NANCY: So what do you want me to do?

THERAPIST: I think it's important for you to promise that should you want to stop treatment, you wait and talk to me before doing anything drastic.

Both of the techniques illustrated above can be used to foster more adaptive functioning over the course of treatment. They also can be used in shorter term contacts in which the focus is dictated by the need to partialize the patient's problems and to intervene quickly in order to help the patient to deal with a life crisis or in gaining control of feelings and behaviors that are interfering with his or her ability to cope effectively.

MASTERSON'S CONFRONTATIVE AND RECONSTRUCTIVE PSYCHOTHERAPIES

In treating borderline patients Masterson (1972, 1976) and Masterson and Rinsley (1975) have described two related approaches based on their view of the role of the split object-relations unit (rewarding and withdrawing), split ego (pleasure and reality), and the pathological defenses against abandonment depression in borderline pathology.

Treatment Goals and Framework

In the beginning stage of work with borderline patients Masterson and Rinsley recommend a confrontative (formerly called supportive) treatment that aims at making the patient's pathological defenses and internalized object relations, which are activated in the transference, ego alien. If successful this approach decreases their self-destructive acting-out and regressive behavior and improves overall functioning. A reconstructive treatment that attempts to work through the patient's abandonment depression and to modify both pathological internalized object relations and the defective ego (Hodis, 1986) can then be used with some individuals. These two therapeutic approaches are not always totally distinct from one another. It may be possible to do some working through of the patient's abandonment depression even in confrontative psychotherapy, and in many instances the patient seems able to benefit from a reconstructive approach from the beginning. Because of the ego syntonic nature of their defenses and self-destructive behavior, however, borderline patients often are not suffering enough or sufficiently motivated to undertake reconstructive treatment initially. This type of psychotherapy may heighten the patient's defenses and lead to premature withdrawal from treatment.

A consistent structure is necessary for carrying out the treatment, along with limit-setting, and, when necessary, hospitalization. This structure helps to contain the patient's self-destructive acting-out if verbal techniques are not sufficient. Optimally, reconstructive psychotherapy requires that the patient be seen a minimum of three times a week. The confrontative approach may be conducted on an once or twice a week basis, but the frequency of sessions needs to be adjusted to the patient's need. The durations of both psychotherapies can be many years, and Masterson underscores the importance of patience in working with the borderline's tenacious resistances and early fixations. In confrontative psychotherapy the transference and therapeutic alliances are usually less intense, and the patient does not gain as much control over his pathological defenses as quickly as in reconstructive psychotherapy.

The Nature of the Therapeutic Relationship

As the borderline patient's split object-relations part units show themselves in the transference, the therapist helps the patient to recognize the nature of his or her pathological internalized object relations and ego structure and to work through any abandonment depression. Masterson, however, also stresses that the therapist must be a real person who maintains a positive attitude toward the patient's individuation, actively supports the patient's appropriate efforts at autonomous behavior, and acknowledges his or her achievements. The therapist also maintains an expectation that the patient will act maturely, and explores with concern those situations in which the patient does not. These qualities provide the patient with a new experience with a "good" object that the patient can internalize to take the place of the "bad" object that rewards regressive, clinging behavior.

The necessity of providing the patient with an experience of a "good" object follows from Mahler's emphasis on the role of actual parenting failures rather than Kernberg's focus on the role of instinctual aggression in the genesis of borderline pathology. Unlike Kernberg, Masterson believes that the therapist has a reparative function and suggests that therapeutic neutrality must give way at times to the therapist's deliberate alliance with, acknowledgement of, and pleasurable reaction to the patient's healthy strivings toward separation-individuation. Both Pine (1985) and the Blancks (1974, 1979), who also worked closely with Mahler, have enlarged upon this concept of using the model of parent–child interactions that foster ego development in the therapeutic process with patients who show severe developmental arrests.

Main Techniques and Principal Features

The problem of the initial stage of all psychotherapy with borderline individuals is the ego syntonic nature of the patient's difficulties. Thus, the presence of the splitting defense, which separates the rewarding and withdrawing object-relations part–units, protects the individual from the feelings of abandonment associated with individuation. At the same time, there is an alliance between the rewarding part–unit and the pleasure or pathological ego that makes the patient feel good at the expense of the reality or healthy ego. The patient has not internalized an object-relations unit in which individuation is rewarded. Efforts at separation–individuation activate the withdrawing part–unit and make the patient feel bad, which, in turn, activates the rewarding part–unit.

In the treatment situation both the rewarding and withdrawing object-relations part–units are mobilized. The transference is based on real experiences with past objects who have become internalized, and the patient alternately projects each of the part–units onto the therapist. Initially, however, it is the pathological alliance between the rewarding part–unit and the pleasure ego that shows itself and is ego syntonic. The patient becomes fearful that therapy will lead to individuation and thus, abandonment, and institutes the rewarding part–unit as a resistance. The patient seeks dependency and may feel good but usually is concurrently acting self-destructively.

The treatment process is divided into three phases: testing (resistance), working through (introject work or definition), and separation (resolution). Distinct conceptually, they often overlap in practice, and so the treatment may go back and forth. While confrontation is the dominant technique in the first stage and communicative matching is used more extensively later in treatment, the therapist must be ready to switch techniques flexibly in all stages. The first stage may last a few months or a few years. It ends with the patient's overcoming of his or her initial resistance and with the concomitant development of a therapeutic alliance. During this period trust in the therapist must be developed, and so the patient tests the therapist repeatedly to see if he or she can withstand the patient's self-destructive behavior without retaliating or withdrawing. In the second, or working through stage, the patient repeatedly replays his or her conflicts around dependency and autonomy over and over in the transference in an effort to avoid a painful depression. The therapeutic alliance that has now consolidated can be used to help the patient understand the nature and origin of his or her internalized difficulties more fully, to gain greater behavioral control, to replace the pathological object-relations unit with a new object-relations unit, and to mourn the past. The final separation phase comes as the patient is able to engage in more autonomous behavior without depression. The impending separation from the therapist renews abandonment fears and mobilizes regressive defenses that need to be worked through. It needs to proceed according to the patient's pace, and the therapist's continuing availability may be important over time.

This treatment process will be illustrated below using the case of Lisa, age 38, who was drinking excessively when she began treatment. Having never realized her ambitions to be an actress, she worked at various secretarial positions that she hated. She still identified herself as an actress but rarely went on auditions or took lessons. She had all but given up her hopes for a theatrical career and was preoccupied with self-loathing and feelings of helplessness and hopelessness. In the past, whatever small successes she had professionally had been followed by depression and self-sabotaging behavior. For example, after getting a role as a rather attractive ingenue on a soap opera, she promptly gained 30 pounds and her limited contract was not renewed. She then moved back in with her parents for a time only to leave to be with a man with whom she had a tortured interaction. Her relationships with men were generally disastrous. She soon became bored by any man who seemed to care for her and had trouble leaving those who mistreated her. Lisa often spent time with her aging parents whom she felt she could not live without, and had failed, despite the fact that they had given her everything. An only child, she felt she had been the center of their lives. She still confided in her mother, who often made her feel worse. She broke her engagement to the one man who wanted to marry her shortly before the wedding, and stayed in a relationship with another who was overtly having an affair with one of her friends. Both fearing and guilty about any kind of autonomous behavior, she was convinced that she would never be successful professionally and would also be alone the rest of her life. More recently she had begun to abuse alcohol to relieve her feelings of depression, but then felt even more self-contempt as a consequence of her drinking. The only time Lisa permitted herself real pleasure was on her annual vacation trips to exotic places on which she showed an unusual sense of adventure, fearlessness, and ingenuity.

Making the Pathological Object-Relations Dynamics Ego Alien

The main objective of confrontative psychotherapy and of the first stage of reconstructive treatment is to make the alliance between the patient's pleasure ego and his or her rewarding part–unit ego alien. This is achieved through "confrontative clarification" of the patient's regressive and clinging behavior, of its destructiveness, and of its defensive role in protecting the patient from feelings of abandonment. The therapist represents reality and opposes the patient's pleasure ego. Since this intervention interferes with the patient's rewarding part–unit and promotes more autonomous behavior, it activates the patient's withdrawing part–unit. The patient no longer feels good even though he or she may be acting more independently. Consequently the patient resists this change and the rewarding part–unit reasserts itself as a defense. The therapist continues to point out and interpret the developments of this circular process involving initial resistance (rewarding part–unit), reality clarification, working through of the feelings of abandonment generated by the withdrawing part–unit, more resistance represented by the reemergence of the rewarding part–unit, further reality clarification, and thus, repeated working through.

From the outset in the treatment of Lisa it seemed clear that her rewarding object-relations unit (RORU) was ego syntonic and needed to be confronted This inevitably led to the activation of her withdrawing object-relations unit (WORU). While she verbalized a wish to be more autonomous, her self concept and almost all of her behavior reflected her active clinging to her depression, dependence, sense of failure, hopelessness, and helplessness. She fought the idea that she could make anything of her life and her treatment sessions showed a resistance to examining her difficulties. Instead, she verbalized her doubts that any therapist could help her and repeatedly considered dropping out of treatment.

LISA: I can't even begin to think about auditioning or getting a better job or dating. It's no use. There's nothing you can do for me. I'm a fuck-up. I didn't even get to the AA meeting I promised myself I would go to. I'm wasting your time.

THERAPIST: This is your way of keeping yourself safe and protecting yourself from any efforts to be independent.

LISA: I don't like being a failure.

THERAPIST: You cling to the idea that you can't do anything. You suffer on the one hand, but this is a more comfortable position for you then is your trying to be more autonomous. It feels better to come in and devalue yourself and be hopeless than to start doing something for yourself.

LISA: I don't know what to do.

THERAPIST: This is the part of you talking that is afraid to be independent. This is the safe position. Being more assertive, or even committing yourself to treatment, is unsafe. Who knows what treatment will lead to?

LISA: Why do you think I need to stay safe?

THERAPIST: I suspect you are being a good girl. You're keeping your mother happy. You're reassuring her that you will never leave her. Even when you reproach yourself you are reassuring her that she doesn't have to worry. You won't go too far from home.

It became clear that Lisa's RORU was based on a deep inner conviction that she was essential to her mother's well being, and on her guilt over abandoning her mother. At the same time her WORU stemmed from her fear that she would destroy her mother if she had her own life. She would be a murderer and wind up alone since no one else would love or take care of her. She had to remain dependent to keep her mother alive, but at the expense of any individuality or real pleasure. The only time she really could get free was on vacation, during which Lisa could show her split off autonomous strivings and competence since it didn't count somehow. It was not part of her day-to-day life. With the therapist's repeated confrontations of Lisa's RORU she became more involved in treatment and took some very small steps in her life, which activated her WORU and in turn, revived her RORU.

LISA: I looked in the trade papers over the weekend and made a list of possible auditions I could go to. I cleaned out my closet and found some clothes that fit that I could wear. I tried them on and then I thought "Who are you kidding? You're no actress."

THERAPIST: You take a step toward doing something for yourself and you get scared and you have to return to your safe position.

LISA: I didn't want to tell you. I've been going to AA and I've been doing okay until yesterday. I slipped. I can't even last a month.

THERAPIST: Why weren't you going to tell me about the slip?

LISA: I thought you would criticize me and tell me that I was wasting your time.

THERAPIST: Who would say that?

LISA: I guess I always think my mother is disappointed in me and thinks I can't do anything right.

THERAPIST: I think you need to keep convincing her that she's right. She has a daughter who is going to be dependent on her forever. You must feel that that's what she really wants and that's what I want, and so you sabotage yourself.

LISA: I feel very depressed. You're making it harder for me to stay the way I am but I don't feel good when I try to mobilize myself.

Developing a Therapeutic Alliance

The process described above allows an alliance to develop between the therapist's and patient's healthy (reality) egos. In order for the therapeutic alliance to solidify the patient must begin to internalize the therapist as a positive external object who supports the patient's individuation without abandoning him or her. The therapeutic alliance can then be used to counter the patient's pathological alliance between his or her rewarding part–unit and pleasure ego, and to induce the patient to give up his or her reliance on the pleasure ego.

LISA: I had a dream that upset me last night. I was at an audition and no one was paying any attention to me. I was speaking and the words stopped coming out. I was talking but I couldn't hear myself.

THERAPIST: Who else was in the dream?

LISA: There were a lot of older people standing around and a woman was sitting off in a corner. Maybe it was you?

THERAPIST: Perhaps it's hard for you to believe that I would be interested in your performance and applaud your success? You fear that I will be like your family and want you to stay dependent on me forever and that I, too, will abandon you if you're independent and happy.

LISA: Now that you mention it, I was afraid to tell you that I've been sober for a month. Yesterday was my anniversary.

THERAPIST: Congratulations. You've worked hard. Why were you reluctant to share that with me?

LISA: I don't know.

THERAPIST: You brought it up when I suggested that you feared I would abandon you if you were more autonomous.

LISA: Yes. I had this strange fear that you would minimize it or ignore it.

THERAPIST: Like in the dream?

LISA: I guess so.

THERAPIST: The relationship with me is threatening and unsafe. If you disobey your mother and listen to me, will I be there or will you be all alone?

Internalization of a New Object-Relations Unit

In those patients who move on to reconstructive psychotherapy the repeated confrontations and interpretations of their pathological internalized object-relations unit make them more aware of their conflicts around individuation. At the same time, their ongoing experience with a therapist who approves of autonomous behavior and who does not abandon them results in the internalization of a new object-relations unit, a constructive self + "good" therapist + "good" feeling or affect. In this phase, as well as in the final ones, when the patient has worked through some of his or her abandonment depression and engages in more individuated behavior, "communicative matching" is an important tool. The therapist actively encourages and approves of the patient's independent wishes and efforts in ways that are similar to the mother's provision of "supplies" to the growing child. Since borderline patients have had little of this type of early experience in which their attempts at individuation have been reacted to positively both verbally and non-verbally, the therapist should provide experiences of this sort. As the patient shows signs of a newly emerging self in the treatment, the therapist conveys interest, enthusiasm, and even a mood and manner similar to that of the patient.

LISA: Rio was fabulous! I can't believe I almost let my mother talk me out of going.

THERAPIST: Tell me about the trip.

LISA: It was just great . . . I didn't want to come back. I'm planning a trip to the Amazon for next year.

THERAPIST: That sounds like fun.

LISA: Well, it's back to the grind now. I've got to get my act together. I got a call on my answering machine yesterday asking me to get in touch with the woman I spoke to about a part before I left. I was excited. I caught myself turning it into something negative and I was able to stop.

THERAPIST: That's quite a victory.

LISA: I think so too.

THERAPIST: Perhaps it's a little dangerous for you to feel too good though?

LISA: You're probably right. I may sabotage myself.

Working Through of Abandonment Depression

The patient's withdrawing part–unit creates painful feelings in the patient as he or she engages in more autonomous behavior. It is necessary for the patient not only to be aware of his or her destructive patterns that develop to ward off these emotions, but also to work through feelings of depression, rage, fear, guilt, passivity, helplessness, and emptiness that are part of his or her abandonment depression. This involves separating from and mourning past internalized objects. This painful process frees the patient of destructive aggression, and the new object-relations unit described above forms the basis of "good" self-representations while the pleasure ego becomes equated with "bad" self-representations. The working through of the patient's abandonment depression and the internalization of a new object-relations unit is accompanied by the patient's increasing ability to differentiate "good" and "bad" self- from "good" and "bad" object-representations, and eventually to develop an integrated conception of self and others.

LISA: I'm very depressed. I've really regressed. I haven't been able to do a thing all week. I really wanted to drink or call that jerk, Alan, who dumped me last year, just to have sex.

THERAPIST: What are your thoughts about why this is happening?

LISA: I had this awful fight with my mother. It wasn't really a fight. I just told her I wasn't going to be able to drive her to a wedding because I had a small part in a play. She didn't even hear me. She just kept acting as if I was being difficult. I got mad and told her that she never supports me when I'm doing what I want to do. She got hurt and started crying. I felt terrible.

THERAPIST: So you wind up sabotaging yourself. You turn your anger at her against yourself.

LISA: I'm mad because I did it to myself. I didn't have to tell her I was in a play. I could have told her that the car was broken and that it had to be fixed.

THERAPIST: I guess you still want her to be happy for you and find it hard to give up the hope that she will come through for you.

LISA: You don't understand how painful it is when I see how I'm disappointing her.

THERAPIST: I think you feel that it really is your job to make her happy and that when you don't succeed it is your fault. You blame yourself as if you are doing something bad, and believe that you will be doomed to a life of aloneness because no one else will ever applaud your success if she doesn't.

LISA: Who else is ever going to care about me? They're not exactly beating down my door. I'm just going to be alone all my life. My parents will die and I'll kill myself.

THERAPIST: Perhaps you feel that your parents have broken their end of the bargain they made with you. If you stay a child forever, they will take care of you forever. Magically, they will never die. Maybe you're enraged that they're getting older because you know they will die and that you will have to be on your own. You've kept your end of the bargain, but they're not going to be able to keep theirs.

LISA: Are you trying to make me feel worse?

THERAPIST: I guess you feel I'm confronting you with a painful reality — that no matter how hard you try to keep them alive by staying a child you won't succeed. In fact, you will have sacrificed yourself in vain.

LISA: I feel like crying. I feel such a sense of loss.

THERAPIST: It is difficult to grieve what you will never have from your mother. Sometimes you try to avoid the pain by going back to your comfortable position. You try to drink your pain away, or sabotage your work, or get involved with someone who mistreats you and distracts you.

LISA: I can't even do those things anymore. You've ruined my ability to escape.

THERAPIST: Perhaps you're angry at me for that.

LISA: Yes. No. I don't know. I think you've helped me.

THERAPIST: It's important for you grieve for what you have not had from your family that isn't your fault so that you can feel free to be your own person without guilt and fear.

Countertransference Issues

Masterson describes three important issues that affect the therapist's countertransference in the treatment of borderline patients: (1) the patient's sensitive awareness of and frequent attacks on the therapist's Achilles' heel in order to test his or her competence, to fulfill pathologic needs, or to resist treatment; (2) the patient's use of projective identification in which both the rewarding and withdrawing object-relations part–units are projected onto the therapist, who begins to feel and sometimes to act in accordance with what is being projected; and (3) the blind spots that stem from therapists' own personality difficulties that lead them to collude with or exacerbate a patient's pathology. Some of the common problems that can occur result from: a therapist who becomes anxious when the patient acts-out because of his or her own reaction formation against such behavior, and who then confronts the patient angrily; a submissive therapist who can never confront the patient's acting out behavior; a dependent therapist who needs the patient's approval and encourages too much regression; a non-directive, passive therapist who stimulates regressive and self-destructive behavior; a directive therapist who blocks autonomous behavior and encourages regressive behavior; or a borderline therapist who distances from, clings to, or alternates between distancing and clinging behavior with the patient.

CONCLUSION

In describing and illustrating the two major conflict-based treatment models this chapter has examined their treatment goals and framework, views of the therapeutic relationship, main techniques and principal features, and outlook on countertransference. It has shown that while Masterson and Rinsley restrict their focus to a narrower range of pathology than does Kernberg, both approaches aim at modifying pathological defenses and internalized object relations through confrontation and interpretation of the transference. Each recommends a consistent and highly structured treatment framework. Both involve normative conceptions about what is desirable behavior and believe that the therapist is an expert observer of objective reality. In contrast to Kernberg, who is adamant about the therapist's maintenance of technical neutrality in expressive psychotherapy, Masterson and Rinsley also see an important role for the therapist as a real person who supports the patient's efforts at individuation. Kernberg's model is unique in its emphasis on the role of aggression, as compared to Masterson and Rinsley's focus on abandonment depression. While both models stress those qualities of therapists that make them vulnerable to countertransference reactions, Kernberg places greater importance on the understanding and use of induced countertransference.

7

Deficit-Based
Treatment Models

In contrast to the conflict-based treatment models of Kernberg and Masterson and Rinsley that were discussed in Chapter 6, this chapter will present examples of three major deficit-based psychotherapeutic approaches. It will describe and illustrate the ego building model of Gertrude and Rubin Blanck, the self psychological treatment of Kohut and his followers, particularly as applied to the treatment of borderline pathology by Bernard Brandchaft and Robert Stolorow, and the mixed approach of Gerald Adler along with his collaborator, Dan Buie, which draws on ego psychology, object relations theory, and self psychology.

THE BLANCKS'S EGO BUILDING
PSYCHOTHERAPY

Arguing that patients with weak egos cannot tolerate certain aspects of traditional psychoanalysis, Gertrude and Rubin Blanck have devised an ego building psychotherapy that is geared specifically to the needs of those borderline individuals who show severe deficits in their ego structure.

Treatment Goals and Framework

Drawing on contemporary ego psychological theory and the work of Hartmann, Spitz, Jacobson, and Mahler, in particular, the Blancks argue that the main goal of their treatment model is to increase the structuralization of the ego directly through a variety of ego building techniques, rather than indirectly through the confrontation and interpretation of internalized object relations. The specific aims of treatment for any given patient are individualized and determined by the therapist's assessment of the patient's particular ego deficits and separation–individuation subphase inadequacies.

While the framework in which psychotherapy is conducted should be clear and consistent, there are few hard-and-fast rules about the frequency of the sessions, the use of a face-to-face or a reclining position, the granting of extra sessions, the degree of the therapist's activity both in and out of the sessions, and the like. The framework should be established in keeping with the therapist's evaluation of a patient's needs and difficulties, rather than on either an arbitrary or inflexible set of guidelines. Important factors in setting the treatment framework are the patient's level of anxiety, degree of motivation, tendency toward regression, degree of primary and secondary process thinking, degree of object constancy, and need for "measured gratifications." The main rule of thumb that guides the choice of techniques is that the less intact the patient the more the treatment will need to vary from classical techniques. While the Blancks indicate that they usually prefer that the patient attends sessions several times a week and sits up, they indicate that psychotherapy can be conducted on an once a week basis, or even less for maintenance, and that the couch can be used in some instances. In their approach the therapist usually must be active in focusing the sessions, flexible in scheduling extra sessions, and willing to provide necessary supports such as postcards during vacation periods or telephone calls between sessions with some patients.

The Nature of the Therapeutic Relationship

Real Object Experiences

Rather than analyzing the transference from a position of technical neutrality as in Kernberg's model, the therapist who uses an ego building approach functions at times as a real rather than a transference object. With those patients who show severe ego deficits the therapist not only provides a benign and caring atmosphere but consciously and deliberately uses his or her relationship with the patient to facilitate ego progression. There are several reasons for this emphasis. First, the process of internalization, which has been faulty in borderline individuals, is fostered by experiences with a therapist who, as a representative of the object world, catalyzes patients' ego development, enables "selective identifications" and reparative work to occur, and helps patients to acquire greater empathy with themselves and with how the object world should have been in their early lives. The therapist selectively replicates the growth enhancing aspects of the parent–child relationship. Second, because less structured borderline patients have not acquired stable internalizations and lack self and object differentiation, they do not always form transferences in the traditional sense. They live in the immediacy of their experience. Through their participation in new, more positive interactions in treatment, they can be helped to move beyond their developmental arrests. Finally, these individuals have difficulties with verbalization and must be permitted to express their needs through action or symbolic means to some degree, while also being simultaneously helped to put their feelings into words rather than actions. While it is important that patients be prevented from engaging in behavior that disrupts the therapeutic relationship, the usual therapeutic rule against action, with its emphasis on having the patient express everything verbally, is too restrictive for those with severe ego deficits (Shane, 1977).

Despite recognizing the importance of real object experiences, the Blancks prefer to engage in more verbal techniques and to serve as catalysts for growth whenever possible, rather than to become participants in the interaction. Measured gratifications should not be provided to every patient or all of the time. They must be used cautiously. They distinguish between what they feel to be their more circumscribed and diagnostically specific view of the role of the therapist as a real object from Alexander's (Alexander & French, 1946) more general conception of the therapist as providing a "corrective emotional experience." They point out that the therapist does not really replace parental functions or provide reparenting per se since one cannot treat an adult the way one would a child, nor is it possible to make up in a direct way for what has or has not happened in the patient's childhood past.

Determining what the patient has missed and how to repair the developmental lesions that exist requires sophisticated, highly attuned assessment skills and creative yet disciplined responses. To the degree that "measured" gratifications are indicated, they should be communicated symbolically in ways that are appropriate to working with adults. For example, with a patient who had severe insomnia related to fears of aloneness and abandonment, one might permit a brief telephone call at night in order to provide a soothing connection (Edward, 1976). Likewise, in a case in which the patient experienced the therapist as so physically distant as to make meaningful communication seem impossible, the therapist might move his or her chair closer to the patient. Other forms of providing measured gratifications involve the self-disclosing of personal information by the therapist, showing an active interest in and enthusiasm for a patient's activities, and using oneself or other transitional objects during periods of separation that are difficult for patients to tolerate. It is not only the therapist's positive human qualities and availability that aid structure building, however, but also his or her recognition and validation of the patient's strengths, ability to set appropriate limits, and provision of growth-enhancing frustrations.

While providing real object experiences when indicated, the therapist must possess an attitude that "guards the autonomy" of the patient and avoids directing the patient's life, using himself or herself as a model of how to live, imposing his or her own values, or encouraging too much dependency. Whatever identifications take place in the treatment as a result of the impact of the therapeutic relationship should be consistent with the patient's innate and developing potentialities. Dependency occurs, of necessity, but it is a temporary way-station on the road to the patient's eventual independence.

The Importance of Positive Transference

With borderline patients who do develop transference reactions, it is important initially to encourage their positive feelings since the borderline patient needs help in overcoming a tendency to be overtaken by negative perceptions of external objects. While transference distortions interfere with the patient's ability to experience the therapist as a good object and should be corrected, too much emphasis on negative reactions before a solid positive transference is established may stimulate unneutralized aggression and threaten to destroy the therapeutic relationship. When patients achieve some degree of separation from internalized negative self- and object-representations, they become freer to respond to the therapist as a real person (Edward, 1976). In order to facilitate this change the therapist must always avoid replicating the pathological parent–child interaction in the treatment.

Main Techniques and Principal Features

Ego support goes far beyond being "nice" to patients and trying to make them feel better. Fortunately there are a vast number of ego building procedures that can be used in the treatment process since the borderline patients' ego deficits are varied and numerous. The following discussion of ego building techniques is only suggestive of the main thrust of the interventions that can be utilized.

Supporting the Ego's Highest Level of Development

Since borderline patients often are unaware of their accomplishments, they lack a sense of mastery and self-esteem. The therapist enhances these ego functions by searching for and pointing out the patient's highest developmental achievements. This is done not in an ingratiating, patronizing, or general way but genuinely, in relation to specific experiences that the patient shares with the therapist. It involves the therapist's ability to listen to the many aspects of a patient's account and to recognize and validate that which represents the patient's most positive attainments, despite the presence of other less optimal behavior.

In the following example the therapist was initially concerned about the patient's anxiety and guilt about having asserted herself and about the somewhat inopportune way in which she had done so. She quickly realized, however, that the patient, who consistently tried to please others at the expense of her even being able to identify let alone gratify her own needs, had taken an important step. Instead of immediately exploring the patient's impulsiveness, abandonment fears, and remorse at this time, the therapist validated the patient's self-assertion.

LISA: I'm a nervous wreck and I've been very down on myself this week.

THERAPIST: Did something happen?

LISA: Nothing special. Well there was something. My mother and I had a scene over the weekend. I've been upset ever since. I wanted to get drunk afterward but I bought a quart of ice cream instead and ate it all. Then I hated myself for having done that and went to sleep early to get away from my feelings.

THERAPIST: Do you want to tell me about the scene?

LISA: I went to visit and have dinner with my mother and I noticed that I was getting irritated from the minute I arrived. First she criticized what I was wearing. She talked incessantly about my cousin's impending marriage and never asked me about my new job. Then she assumed that I was going to drive her to the country next week so that she could visit her sister. I told her that I couldn't because of another commitment that I had. She wouldn't listen to me. I don't know how I stood my ground but I did. I said that I was sorry but that I couldn't do it. So then she said I was selfish and said that she couldn't understand what I had to do that was so important. I lost it. I started crying and walked out and slammed the door.

THERAPIST: I can see why you were upset. Is that when you wanted to drink?

LISA: Yes. I felt terrible and thought of going back but I just went home. I stopped to buy some ice cream.

THERAPIST: It seems important that you were able to recognize that you did not want to drive her to the country, had a right to follow through with your own plans, and that you asserted yourself with her.

LISA: I actually felt good about it too but then I started to feel frightened and guilty. I almost called her back to say I had changed my plans but something wouldn't let me do it.

THERAPIST: It took courage to take the risk of not calling her back.

LISA: I do feel a little stronger. I wish I didn't feel as if I had done a terrible thing. I feel like a bad girl who doesn't love her mother.

THERAPIST: This is a very familiar feeling that you have when your needs seem to conflict with someone else's needs. But at least you are beginning to stand up for yourself.

In the next vignette, Ron, who had left numerous therapists previously without ever telling them he was angry, startled the current therapist with the intensity of his rage and distortions. The therapist was able to recognize, however, that Ron had come for his session despite his anger and was openly showing his feelings rather than acting them out by prematurely terminating or staying away from treatment. Rather than pointing out Ron's "inappropriate" reactions or exploring the extent of his rage, the therapist commented on the more adaptive behavior Ron showed in coming to the session.

RON: Last week you cut my session time short! Who do you think you are? I think you are a money hungry and totally callous person. I'm tired of your ripping me off. You must really get off on your power.

THERAPIST: I wasn't aware of cutting the session short, but even if I had done that, I'm puzzled as to why you would think I did it intentionally or to exploit you?

RON: Don't give me that crap. If you weren't aware of it, that's even worse. Are you brain damaged? Maybe you're developing Alzheimer's disease. My watch said I had 2 minutes left.

THERAPIST: I'm sorry that you feel so cheated by me and we need to talk more about this, but I think it's important that you were able to confront me personally with your complaint rather than stay away from the session. You took a risk.

RON: I wasn't going to come back. I was going to write you off. I'm not even sure why I'm here.

THERAPIST: I know it has been difficult for you in the past to tell your therapists when they have disappointed or angered you, and you have left them instead of verbalizing your feelings directly to them.

RON: So I'm verbalizing my feelings. What are you going to do about it?

THERAPIST: If you feel I ended the session too early I will make up the time today, but I think we should talk more about your feeling that I'm money grubbing and ripping you off.

Improving the Defensive Function of the Ego

Most borderline patients lack the ability to recognize when and under what conditions they become anxious. Likewise, they do not cope with their anxiety adaptively, and utilize primitive defenses or engage in behavior that has negative consequences. Rather than confront and interpret the patient's defenses and behavior, the therapist can help the patient to understand the process by which they become anxious and potentially self-destructive and to find more effective ways of soothing themselves or dealing with the anxiety provoking stimuli or situations. This can take quite a lot of active effort, as is shown in the example below.

JEFF: I was driving my motorcycle last night and the police stopped me and gave me a ticket. The creep said I was speeding. I wanted to punch him out. I think he saw that I was ready to explode and he backed off. It's a good thing. If he had made one sarcastic comment I might have let him have it. This is all I needed. I already have points against me. I was almost in an accident last month. I may lose my license.

THERAPIST: Were you actually speeding?

JEFF: I was going pretty fast even for me. I just didn't care.

THERAPIST: It seems that you must have been feeling quite upset about something to be putting yourself at risk.

JEFF: I wasn't feeling anything other than that I wanted to go as fast as possible. I knew I shouldn't have but I just wanted to do it.

THERAPIST: Usually when you do something that is self-defeating, it comes after you have felt rejected or demeaned. It's hard for you to feel painful emotions and you try to blot them out.

JEFF: I can't think of anything.

THERAPIST: It is important that we try to understand what you were experiencing. What happened during the day?

JEFF: It was a usual day. After I left your office I went to work.

THERAPIST: How did you feel when you left here?

JEFF: Why are you asking?

THERAPIST: I'm wondering if you became upset by something that happened in the session and whether these feelings are connected to your speeding?

JEFF: You're always trying to make connections like that.

THERAPIST: You're right. I do that to help you identify what you are feeling so that you can learn to cope with your reactions in more constructive ways. Sometimes you don't recognize what upsets you or even that you are disturbed. Is it possible you were angry with me yesterday?

JEFF: Well now that you ask, I remember that you seemed sleepy. I thought you weren't paying attention to me.

THERAPIST: Tell me more about what that was like for you.

JEFF: I felt empty when I left the session. I didn't feel like going to work. I kept thinking that I wanted to take my motorcycle out for a ride. Maybe you're right. Maybe I had to get away from what I was feeling.

THERAPIST: There's nothing wrong with trying to help yourself to feel better but when you try to blot out your feelings, they often express themselves in your doing something to hurt yourself. Perhaps you're wanting to punch out the policeman was related to your loss of connection with me and your feeling that I didn't care about you?

JEFF: I'm just a patient. Why should you care?

Encouraging Positive Affective Connections

Borderline individuals often lack an inner experience of stable connections to positive objects, and are filled with angry affects that weaken whatever positive bonds they have. Their unneutralized aggression makes them feel more alone. Particularly in the initial stage of treatment, the therapist should be cautious in encouraging the ventilation of angry feelings or in drawing attention either to patients' rage at key people in their lives or to their emptiness. Instead, the therapist should reinforce the positive connections to people that exist until the capacity for neutralization is somewhat developed and the patient, despite his or her anger, is able to maintain good feelings towards others.

In early sessions with Lisa it was clear that her idealization of and devotion to her mother masked intense rage. Whenever Lisa experienced any irritation at her mother she also experienced a total sense of aloneness and became guilt-ridden and self-destructive. Instead of dealing with this dynamic or probing for Lisa's anger at her mother initially, the therapist was careful to emphasize the caring aspects of Lisa's relationship with her mother. She did not feel that the therapeutic relationship with Lisa was sufficiently strong at this time to enable Lisa to explore her rage without overwhelming feelings of guilt and aloneness.

LISA: Sometimes I find myself wanting to scream in my mother's presence and then I feel like killing myself. Something minor will set it off. If she so much as implies that I'm not doing enough for her I get very upset.

THERAPIST: It hurts you a lot when your mother does not appreciate how devoted you are to her.

LISA: She thinks I don't care at all.

THERAPIST: You do a great deal to try to make her life more comfortable.

LISA: When she tells me that I'm selfish I begin to believe it and hate myself and her at the same time. I know it's stupid.

THERAPIST: It's important to remember at those times how important her well-being has been to you and how much you have done to try to meet her needs.

Aiding Verbalization

Because of their ongoing symbiotic longings, many borderline individuals wish to be understood without having to communicate their thoughts and feelings. Their difficulty in verbalization may result from either too much or too little gratification early in their lives. When a patient has been overindulged symbiotically, the therapist holds out the expectation that the patient try to communicate verbally and helps the patient do so. In instances where the patient has been deprived of a comfortable symbiosis it may be necessary for the therapist to respond to the patient's nonverbal requests or communications to some degree. The ultimate goal, however, is to strengthen the patient's ability to verbalize and thereby to bring the patient's preverbal experiences under the control of the ego. Verbalization replaces or at least postpones action.

Different phases of the work with Jeff, who had been physically abused by his mother and neglected by his father, illustrates both of these strategies. Jeff had never been able to turn to anyone for nurturing as a child and often was in the position of parenting both his mother and father. Compliant at home, he was rebellious at school and often got into trouble. As an adult he tried to be a lawyer but felt unsuccessful and ungratified. Jeff was also quite self-destructive in his personal as well as his professional life.

On the one hand he never expected anyone to be there for him. On the other hand he had intense longings to be totally understood and cared for without his having to say or do anything. The therapist learned that Jeff often left sessions feeling empty and depressed. He had lost his sense of connection to the therapist, but never called to touch base. Out of touch with his feelings, he often would act-out. On one of the numerous occasions when the therapist sensed that Jeff was upset upon leaving the session he called Jeff to find out how he was. Both surprised and moved by the therapist's reaching out to him in this way, Jeff gradually began to feel closer to the therapist and was able to maintain himself between sessions without acting-out, but still had difficulty getting in touch with and verbalizing his feelings when they occurred. On one occasion the therapist noticed that Jeff seemed agitated and withdrawn at the end of their session and invited Jeff to stay a few minutes longer and urged him to talk about what he was experiencing.

JEFF: I just want to leave. I don't know what I'm feeling.

THERAPIST: I know it's hard for you but I think it's important for you to try to say what's going on for you before you leave.

JEFF: You probably know what's wrong. Why do you have to have me say it?

THERAPIST: I can see something is bothering you but I really don't know what it is. I need you to help me out.

JEFF: I just feel empty.

THERAPIST: Perhaps you can take a minute to think about what is upsetting you?

JEFF: I feel you're playing a game with me.

THERAPIST: I'm not trying to do that. I just can't read your mind. It seems to happen to you a lot. You leave here upset but are unable to tell me what's bothering you.

JEFF: I don't want to give you the satisfaction of knowing that you hurt me. I'm not sure why I said that. I don't really feel that you hurt me.

THERAPIST: Maybe I did and it's hard for you to acknowledge that I'm important enough to you to have hurt you.

JEFF: I just don't think you pay attention to me sometimes. You don't seem to remember the things I tell you.

THERAPIST: What did I seem not to remember today?

JEFF: Today's my birthday.

THERAPIST: I didn't know that.

JEFF: Well, I didn't really tell you but I somehow thought you would know. I guess I do that a lot.

THERAPIST: How are you feeling now?

JEFF: I feel a little better.

THERAPIST: Do you have plans to celebrate?

JEFF: I'm going out with friends.

THERAPIST: I hope you have a Happy Birthday.

Differentiation of Affects and Help with Other Regulatory Processes

Often having affect storms or becoming flooded by intense rage, borderline individuals generally have difficulty discriminating among their feelings. The therapist can focus specifically on enabling patients to recognize and differentiate their distinct affects and to verbalize their feelings, as is shown in the following example.

JEFF: I'm beginning to realize that I'm angry most of the time. I go around feeling either empty or filled with hatred for everyone.

THERAPIST: Perhaps sometimes it is easier for you to be angry than to experience other emotions that make you feel more vulnerable?

JEFF: Like what?

THERAPIST: Sadness, loneliness, longing, affection, hurt. Let's look at what happened the other day when I didn't know it was your birthday.

JEFF: I know what you're going to say. You're going to tell me that you can't be expected to read my mind.

THERAPIST: I wasn't going to say that. I was going to ask you to try to pinpoint what you were feeling a little more. There are many different reactions that you might have had that led you to feel empty and depressed.

JEFF: I just felt let down.

THERAPIST: Tell me a little more about what you're feeling right now.

JEFF: I never had a birthday party when I was a kid. I used to hope that my parents would surprise me. They never did.

THERAPIST: You look sad.

JEFF: Do I? Maybe I am. I don't like to feel sad. Sometimes I wish . . .

THERAPIST: What do you wish for?

JEFF: I'd like to know you a little better. I don't know anything about you. I don't know if you're married or have children. I guess I feel left out.

THERAPIST: You've never really asked me any personal questions.

JEFF: I thought you wouldn't answer them.

THERAPIST: Then you would feel more left out.

JEFF: It doesn't seem fair. Our relationship is very one-sided.

THERAPIST: You felt that a lot with your own parents.

JEFF: That's for sure.

Promoting Exercise of Function

The therapist helps patients to think and do for themselves, thereby exercising and developing mastery of their own abilities. Whenever possible it is better to have patients arrive at their own understanding of themselves and to problem solve (as the therapist does below), than to have the therapist give them pronouncements or solutions.

JEFF: I don't want to be self-destructive. I just feel driven sometimes to act. I don't think about what I'm doing and why. I know you say I should get in touch with what's bothering me but I can't stand some of the feelings that I have. I don't know how to deal with them better. Tell me what to do, and I'll try to do it.

THERAPIST: I think you can discover that for yourself. Let us say you're feeling very sad. What do you think you might do to help you to feel better? What might work?

JEFF: Other than riding my motorcycle?

THERAPIST: Riding your motorcycle has been quite a problem lately.

JEFF: I don't really think it's a good idea for me to drive when I'm upset. It's too tempting to speed. It's like going to a bar if you're an alcoholic.

THERAPIST: It's important that you can recognize that. Can you think of a substitute?

JEFF: Maybe I can go to the gym and work out. I usually feel energized when I do something physical.

THERAPIST: Perhaps you could try it and see how it feels. We can talk about the results of your experiment.

Using Confrontation, Explanation, and Interpretation

The Blancks generally recommend the use of explanation and a specific type of ego interpretation over confrontation and more traditional types of interpretation. Confrontation helps the patient's observing ego to look at aspects of the patient's feelings and behavior that he or she may not fully recognize but which are observable. Usually this technique is used later in the treatment. Early on it may stimulate too much unneutralized aggression and disrupt the therapeutic relationship. Explanation, a technique that precedes interpretation, is designed to help the patient understand where, in the developmental process of separation–individuation, he or she developed difficulties. The therapist, who is attuned to the patient's subphase inadequacies, educates the patient about the origins and manifestations of his or her early lesions. This technique is useful in appealing to the patient's observing ego and in making the patient an ally in the process of understanding his or her problems and distortions.

LISA: I don't know why I'm feeling so anxious and guilty. All I did was tell my mother that I'm not driving her to see her sister. I'm 38 years old. I should be able to spend one weekend away from my family.

THERAPIST: It is difficult for you to assert yourself without feeling that you are rejecting and destroying your mother, and that therefore she will abandon you and you will be all alone in return.

LISA: I don't know why I get so frightened. My mother was there for me most of the time.

THERAPIST: I think you had repeated experiences as a child when you were not encouraged to become autonomous, and so believed that your mother wanted you to be dependent on her. You never learned to be on your own and you became fearful that being independent would lead her to abandon you. This belief has carried over into your adult relationships and work life.

Classical interpretations of the genetic (developmental) origins of unconscious wishes and the superego conflicts related to them, as well as transference interpretations, usually should not be made in the treatment of patients with severe ego deficits until the ego has been strengthened. While in many instances the patient's need for the therapist to function as a real object takes precedence over the use of any type of interpretation, there are *ego interpretations* that can be used for the purposes of ego building. In the psychotherapy of patients with severe developmental arrests, tactful and tentatively offered interpretations that are attuned to the most advanced level of what is being expressed should always take precedence over interpretations of conflict-bound resistances.

In making effective interpretations the therapist must distinguish between the adaptive features of the patient's personality that can be used to foster development and those that are maladaptive. The therapist must differentiate pathological defenses and character traits from those aspects of the patient's behavior that are phase appropriate given the patient's developmental level, or which are necessary to preserve the integrity of the ego, as well as behavior that is in the service of growth. For example, wanting to take a vacation from treatment may reflect the patient's positive although uncomfortable efforts to individuate, or may signal the patient's need to draw back from a too intense dependency in order to reassure himself or herself of his or her separateness. Interpreting this request as defensive or evidence of resistance may be experienced by the patient as a lack of attunement and may have a countertherapeutic effect.

In the following example the therapist realized that Lisa was threatened by her increasing assertiveness, which activated her fear of object loss. She was retreating temporarily in order to reassure herself that her dependent needs would be met so that she could go forward again. Instead of exploring and interpreting Lisa's behavior as indicative of her resistance to independence, the therapist interpreted the adaptive aspects of her actions.

LISA: I know you'll be disappointed in me. I spent the weekend with my parents and I chauffeured my mother around. I didn't get a chance to do any research on my new part. I'm annoyed with myself for retreating to my little girl position.

THERAPIST: Maybe it was necessary for you to do that.

LISA: What do you mean?

THERAPIST: Perhaps you needed to connect with your mother in the old way to reassure yourself that she was still there. It seems important to you to know that if you assert yourself, you haven't lost her totally.

LISA: That makes me feel a little better.

Supporting the Developmental Thrust

The therapeutic climate, the provision of ego support and real object experiences, the emphasis on verbalization rather than action, and the patient's exercise of his or her own functions can, over time, develop the patient's internal structure that contributes to the improvement of the regulatory processes and the neutralization of aggression. Since aggression can be used in the service of growth when it is neutralized, the patient gradually moves on to greater developmental achievements. The therapist must recognize and support the patient's steps toward separation–individuation. These initial pushes toward increasing assertiveness and autonomy often are expressed awkwardly or even angrily. It is easy to misinterpret these moves as signs of resistance and to fail to support the patient's positive developmental thrusts. The therapist in the following example initially did this, but then corrected her error.

LISA: I'm excited about a new part I got. It's small but it's meaty. I really went all out to get it. I did a really great audition. Unfortunately, rehearsals are going to interfere with my sessions and I think I'm going to have to miss 2 weeks of treatment.

THERAPIST: Had you thought of asking me to reschedule the times? You know that's my usual policy.

LISA: I just don't see how I'm going to have the time right now.

THERAPIST: I wonder why you arranged your schedule that way?

LISA: Do you really expect me to turn a good part down? I thought you were trying to help me be more successful.

THERAPIST: We have been working toward that but I'm wondering if your wanting to stop sessions for a few weeks represents some anger at me.

LISA: I wasn't upset when I came in but I am now. I thought you would be pleased that I got the part and that I feel strong enough to go without seeing you for a few weeks.

THERAPIST: I can see your point. I guess it is important for you to feel that you can be on your own without feeling that I will be angry or hurt or try to hold you back. In fact, that's quite an achievement for you.

LISA: I'm glad you said that.

THERAPIST: I am still concerned though about the session times that you will miss since we agreed that you would be responsible for the time.

LISA: I can see that. Maybe I can make up the time later.

Patients are also likely to experience regressive pulls and seem to request more dependent gratification as they move forward. The therapist helps the patient to understand these swings but sometimes imposes growth-promoting frustration that furthers the separation–individuation process.

LISA: I need your advice. I don't know what to do about my career. I've been thinking I should really go to California where there are more opportunities for work. I would only stay a few months while they're casting.

THERAPIST: What is your concern about doing that?

LISA: I'm worried I'm not good enough. I'm afraid I'll feel alone. I'm concerned about my mother. I need you to tell me what I should do.

THERAPIST: You have been making your own decisions, and doing pretty well at that, for a while now.

LISA: I just feel scared this time. It's a big step. I want to know you won't be angry and that I can see you when I come back.

THERAPIST: What makes you think I wouldn't see you?

LISA: What should I do? Can I have an extra session this week?

THERAPIST: I can understand your wanting my support and you have it, but do you need to have an extra appointment to convince yourself that I am here and you will not be abandoned? You can handle this decision.

Avoiding Object Replication and Correcting Distortions

The provision of a reliable, consistently benign climate and the absence of counterhostility in the face of negative affects eventually help patients to recognize that the wider object world represented by the therapist is different from the world of primary objects with whom the patient continues to interact (whether or not they are still present). In addition to avoiding the replication of patients' early traumatic interactions with parental figures, the therapist as a real object provides experiences that help the patient acquire new internalizations. Explanation and interpretation of the patient's distortions and of the ways in which early experiences are continuously repeated for the purpose of retention of the patient's original object connections, no matter how negative they were, are important. This can be seen in the following example.

JEFF: I feel like a total fool. I was beginning to trust that you cared about me but I see that you only seem to care when it suits you. You don't give a damn about me. You do what you need to do to keep me coming here and paying you.

THERAPIST: What is making you feel that way?

JEFF: I won an important case and you didn't even call me up to congratulate me.

THERAPIST: How would I know that you had won the case?

JEFF: You knew about the trial. I told you about it. You could have called to see how it turned out.

THERAPIST: I think you are experiencing me right now as you felt with your father who really didn't care. It's hard for you to believe that I would be pleased with your success. You are turning me into your father instead who would either ignore or demean you. By doing that you don't have to leave him behind. He's right there with you telling you that you'll never amount to anything. This has happened before between us when things have gone your way.

JEFF: You're saying I'm distorting your motives.

THERAPIST: Why would I not be interested in your success? What have we been working toward?

JEFF: It feels like you are him sometimes and I hate you.

THERAPIST: This is an internal script that you play out. It represents your relationship with your father which is hard to give up.

Countertransference Issues

The main challenge to therapists in freeing themselves from counter-therapeutic countertransference reactions to borderline patients stems from the impact of these patients' separation–individuation subphase inadequacies on the therapist. Particularly difficult to manage therapeutically are: (1) their compelling needs for narcissistic supplies and their efforts to induce the therapist to replicate their early pathological interactions with significant others; (2) the requirement that the therapist respond to rather than analyze the patient's needs in growth-promoting ways; and (3) the shifting and multiple roles in which the patient casts the therapist. The therapist's use of himself or herself as a real object is relatively uncharted territory as therapists traditionally have practiced an "objective detachment." Little is written to guide a more involved approach (Shane, 1977; Stewart, 1985). Likewise, a therapist's own self knowledge and resolution of his or her own subphase issues may be limited and his or her blind spots can affect the treatment negatively. Since the treatment of the borderline patient's ego deficits necessitates that the therapist provide an experiential interaction with the patient, it is essential that the therapist understand his or her own subphase adequacies and inadequacies so that counter-therapeutic responses can be avoided.

KOHUT AND OTHERS' SELF PSYCHOLOGICAL PSYCHOTHERAPY

Self psychology represents a major departure from classical psycho-analysis, ego psychology, and object-relations theory. Kohut (1971, 1977) developed self psychology to address the problems of individuals with narcissistic disorders, which he and others have differentiated from more severe borderline conditions. Although somewhat pessimistic about the efficacy of his approach with borderline individuals (Kohut, 1984), others, particularly Bernard Brandchaft and Robert Stolorow (1984a, 1984b), have used self psychology successfully with this population.

Treatment Goals and Framework

The goal of self psychological treatment is to help patients to develop a greater degree of self- cohesion. The therapeutic regression that occurs in the treatment process enables patients to reexperience and understand their frustrated selfobject needs for mirroring, idealization, and twinship in a new and more empathic context. The therapist immerses himself or herself in the patient's inner world and intervenes in ways that help patients to make sense of their own subjective truth rather than the therapist's perception of reality. Enabling patients to "experience" rather than only "acquire" knowledge of the self is necessary to the relief of their emotional suffering. It firms up the self and improves the quality of life. Through empathic understanding, optimal frustration, and the repair of disruptions in the selfobject transferences that develop, transmuting internalizations occur that lead to new and stronger self structures. In discussing the nature of therapeutic change, Kohut (1984, p. 77) wrote: "Increased ability to verbalize, broader insight, greater autonomy of ego functions, and increased control over impulsiveness may accompany these gains, but they are not the essence of cure . . . the essence of the psychoanalytic cure resides in the patient's newly acquired ability to identify and seek out appropriate selfobjects — both mirroring and idealizable — as they present themselves in his realistic surroundings and to be sustained by them."

An empathic therapeutic climate is the *sine qua non* of the therapy. The exact details of the structure that is established are less vital than their usefulness in achieving the proper ambience. The specific framework of the treatment with respect to the frequency of sessions, fees, the patient's use of the couch or a face-to-face position, and other practical arrangements is a backdrop against which the patient is helped to revive his or her arrested selfobject needs in the transference. They will vary with the needs of a particular patient. While more frequent sessions and the use of the couch may intensify the therapeutic regression that takes place, this can be positive or negative depending on the individual. A patient must be able to tolerate the regression involved in the selfobject transferences without irreversible fragmentation or severe transference disruptions that interfere with the treatment.

In this approach, being a real person with human qualities is more important than preserving a sterile image in the name of therapeutic neutrality. In this regard, Wolf (1988) argues that therapists' traditional practice of refraining from decorating their offices in keeping with their tastes and interests so as not to reveal too much of themselves actually can inhibit rather than facilitate the development of patients' selfobject transferences and the strengthening of their self expression. Likewise, the goal of helping patients to experience themselves more fully often requires flexibility rather than rigidity in the treatment framework. Rather than set firm limits on patients the therapist needs "to tolerate, often for long periods, seemingly 'crazy' behavior" (Magid, 1984, p. 102).

The Nature of the Therapeutic Relationship

"Experience-Near-Empathy"

Empathy is the main tool for collecting data about the patient. Rather than function as an objective, neutral, and detached observer who makes interpretations from an "experience-distant" position, the therapist engages in "experience-near-empathy" (Kohut, 1959, 1982, 1984). Trying to understand the patient's inner world by a form of "vicarious introspection," in which attempts are made to feel what it is like to be the patient, the therapist does not give his or her view of external reality priority over the patient's subjective experience. Because Kohut believes that it is not possible to observe the patient from a totally objective position since the observer always participates in the interaction to some degree, he regards what occurs in the treatment as a function of the mutual impact of patient and therapist, rather than of the patient's personality only. Thus, the patient's reactions in the treatment, even when seemingly irrational, must be understood in relationship to the therapist's characteristics, behavior, or lack of attunement.

Responding to the question of whether his type of empathy is different than that employed in other non-self psychological therapies, Kohut (1984) indicates that self psychological theory enables the therapist to enlarge and alter his or her perceptions about what is significant to the patient. Thus, the therapist becomes better able to be empathic with the patient's troubling or puzzling reactions and their origins. Maintaining an empathic attitude is particularly difficult, however, in the treatment of borderline individuals whose difficulties in sustaining selfobject transferences result in severe and sometimes unrelenting attacks on the therapist, or who undergo turbulent disruptions of their selfobject ties. It requires a persistent, accepting, self-scrutinizing therapist, who is dedicated to trying to understand the patient despite the narcissistic injuries to which the therapist is exposed by the patient's pathology.

The Selfobject Transferences

The original impetus for self psychology stemmed from Kohut's treatment of patients who did not seem to develop the classical psychoanalytic transferences in treatment, and who did not respond well to traditional types of drive-related interpretations. He observed that these patients related to him in characteristic ways that he interpreted as special types of transference paradigms associated with narcissistic pathology. These narcissistic transferences represented a revival of the patients' frustrated, archaic, selfobject needs for idealization, mirroring, a twin or alter-ego merger, a supportive adversary, or a creative partner. (These were discussed in Chapter 4.) In fact, Kohut diagnosed narcissistic disorders on the basis of whether selfobject transferences developed in the therapeutic relationship. Self psychological treatment permits these transferences to emerge. The therapist then focuses on helping patients to understand their needs and the impact of parenting failures on their current feelings and behavior. The repair of disruptions in the transference leads to greater self-cohesion, more mature selfobject needs, and greater avenues for adult gratification.

Optimal Frustration versus Optimal Responsiveness

Does the self psychological therapist only provide empathic understanding or does he or she attempt to gratify some of the needs that patients express? For example, if the patient wants to be soothed or admired, does the therapist show that he or she recognizes these wishes or does the therapist actually calm or praise the patient? There are differences of opinion within self psychology about whether and when the therapist should selectively meet the patient's needs. Wolf (1988) argues that the emphasis on gratification stems from a misconception about Kohut's intent and strongly favors a more conservative position. Originally, Kohut distinguished between empathy and acts of kindness or sympathy. He felt that a certain amount of optimal frustration was necessary for patients to develop new or stronger internal self structures. Consequently, he did not advise the therapist to deliberately attempt to gratify the patient. Yet, there are repeated instances in Kohut's writings in which he responded to what he felt the patient needed at particular times, and he acknowledged that empathic understanding, in itself, is gratifying. Moreover, as Bacal (1985) points out, Kohut's and others' emphasis on frustration as a prerequisite for the development of psychic structure is an unfortunate carry-over from classical psychoanalysis.

Studies of child development suggest that positive experiences themselves also promote identification and internalization and build the ego or self. White and Weiner (1986) are among those self psychologists who take a more positive view of the role of gratification.

They advocate that therapists fulfill certain selfobject functions. Likewise, Bacal (1985, p. 225) recommends that therapists provide a more conscious, diagnostically specific form of "optimal responsiveness" that encompasses optimal frustration and optimal gratification as indicated. In describing the qualities of gifted therapists, Kohut (1984, p. 170–171) states that "whatever their consciously held and openly professed theoretical beliefs — [they] have always, subtly or not so subtly, discarded their straitlaced reserve in responding to those patients who, during childhood, were deprived of the emotional palpability of the selfobject. And they have thus provided for these patients . . . that minimum of emotional responsiveness without which the analytic work could not proceed optimally."

Empathy as a Corrective Emotional Experience

Does the therapist consciously try to reparent the patient? Kohut advised against the therapist deliberately attempting to play roles that are opposite to those of the parents, and did not believe that treatment makes up for the psychological traumas of the past. Further, even an empathic therapist is not perfect and disappoints and frustrates patients at times (Wolf, 1988, p. 104). Nevertheless, the revival of stunted needs in the transference, which are understood and responded to with empathy, and the repair of whatever disruptions occur, result in transmuting internalizations that give patients a second chance to complete their development and to attain more self- cohesion. While not directly suggesting that therapists provide reparenting, Kohut acknowledged the curative impact of empathy in its own right. Likewise, by emphasizing the importance of the empathic climate and interactive process of the treatment, rather than the content of interpretations, per se, Kohut recognized the power of reparative experiences. Although he was previously reluctant to use the term "corrective emotional experience" because of its association with Alexander's seemingly more manipulative approach that had fallen into disrepute in psychoanalytic circles, in his last book Kohut (1984) embraced a more circumscribed view of this concept.

Valuing the Uniqueness of the Self

The self psychological therapist prizes nondestructive self expression in all its forms rather than a "maturity morality" in which the patient is encouraged to live his or her life in accordance with society's or the therapist's values and expectations regarding what is normal and appropriate. Being different is not equated with being pathological.

This attitude is particularly important in helping patients to find sustaining selfobjects and in expressing their creativity. Enabling the patient to develop "a sense of inner freedom, of joyful search, and the courageous ability to go one's own way" (Kohut, 1984, p. 169) takes precedence over helping them to conform to reality.

Main Techniques and Principal Features

Overcoming Resistances to Selfobject Transferences

An atmosphere of acceptance and empathy spontaneously mobilizes a selfobject transference so that the therapist does not have to induce such a development. However, even higher-functioning narcissistic patients bring fears of varying intensity to the therapeutic relationship and may defend against the emergence of their frustrated childhood needs. The greater their earlier trauma, the more likely it is that they will be frightened of exposing themselves to being disappointed or mistreated once more. Overcoming this "resistance," or "fear of being traumatically injured again" (Wolf, 1988, p. 111), is the main therapeutic task in the initial stage of treatment. The therapist conveys empathic understanding of the nature and reasons for this so-called resistance to the emerging transference. For example, with a patient who repeatedly comes late to early sessions and who seems to be having difficulty sharing feelings, the therapist might comment on the understandable fear the patient might be feeling about coming to rely on the therapist when he or she has never been able to count on anyone in the past.

When selfobject transferences develop, the therapist does not interpret them as evidence of primitive, pathological defenses since they are viewed as positive developments. Thus, when a patient who initially comes late for sessions and does not share feelings easily begins to arrive promptly, talk readily, and show an idealizing transference, the therapist does not attempt to point out, minimize, or reject the idealization, nor does he or she interpret the idealization as a defense against the aggression that must be lurking close by.

Borderline individuals show special problems in forming stable selfobject transferences. In many instances they maintain whatever cohesion they have by avoiding close relationships. For this reason Kohut initially was quite pessimistic about their self psychological treatment. He shifted his position on this point and came to feel they could be helped by the right therapist, who could be empathic with their severe difficulties. Despite their optimism about the treatability of borderline patients, Brandchaft and Stolorow acknowledge that the selfobject ties of these patients are "more primitive and intense, more labile and vulnerable to disruption, and therefore more taxing of the therapist's empathy and tolerance. . . . Furthermore, when the selfobject ties . . . are obstructed or ruptured by empathic failures or separations, the patient's reactions may be much more catastrophic and disturbed" (1984a, p. 344). Nevertheless, they observe that when these patients' compelling, archaic needs for idealization, mirroring of their grandiosity and exhibitionism, and their tumultuous reactions to failures in attunement are understood and responded to sensitively, borderline patients become more accessible and develop intense positive transferences.

Martin, a 34-year-old unemployed actor, fluctuated in early sessions between being overly self-confident and somewhat grandiose and being sullen and withdrawn. In the former instances he would boast of his creative talents and negate the abilities of his more successful peers. In the latter cases he would be noncommunicative or disparaging of the treatment. While the therapist initially experienced Martin's changing states as coming "out of the blue" and was tempted to point out his contradictory behavior, she explored instead Martin's experience of her. When it appeared as if Martin was distorting their interaction based on his past relationships, the therapist refrained from interpreting his "negative transference" and alternatively tried to relate empathically to his needs and fears.

MARTIN: I don't feel like talking today. In fact, I really didn't want to come here. I don't think treatment can work for me.
THERAPIST: Did something happen to make you feel that way?
MARTIN: No. Nothing.
THERAPIST: I wonder how you have been feeling about me?
MARTIN: You've been okay so far.
THERAPIST: So far?
MARTIN: I know you're going to get tired of listening to me.
THERAPIST: What have I done to communicate that?
MARTIN: I know I felt like an idiot after I left the session last week. I was going on about my career and I was thinking that you probably thought I would never amount to anything.
THERAPIST: There haven't been too many people in your life whom you felt were in your corner.
MARTIN: I never could please my parents, especially my father.
THERAPIST: You would naturally like me to be interested in you and you fear that I, like your father, won't care.
MARTIN: I get frightened of you sometimes when I think that way.

THERAPIST: It's understandable that you would feel that you don't want to take the risk of sharing your feelings with me at those times. Given your past experience, it is hard for you to believe that I will be different from others in your life.

MARTIN: Sometimes I begin to think that you are interested and then I find myself closing down. I don't even know why it happens.

THERAPIST: It's hard to believe that someone might care and then find out that you were wrong. Who would want to expose himself to that disappointment?

MARTIN: When you say things like that I feel you understand me.

THERAPIST: But feeling understood makes you feel more vulnerable and so you then try to push me away to protect yourself.

As the treatment went on, Martin's changing states continued in even more dramatic ways. In one session he would seek reassurance and praise from the therapist, and in the next session be argumentative, provocative, and report having used cocaine several times during the week to relieve his depression. The therapist was greatly concerned about Martin's self-destructiveness and considered trying to set a limit on his acting-out. She decided, however, to try first to see if helping Martin to move into a more stable mirror transference would help him to contain his behavior.

MARTIN: I had some really great experiences on coke this week. That stuff is better than therapy. It costs a lot, though, but at least I get something for my money.

THERAPIST: It seems like you feel that I'm not there for you.

MARTIN: Of course you're there. You sit in your chair and you listen and sometimes you smile and nod at the right times. You really have a great technique. You should have gone into acting.

THERAPIST: Do you feel I'm playing a role with you?

MARTIN: You are acting! I'm not saying that you have bad motivations. You probably want to help me but you act as if you are interested and concerned about me and I don't think you are any more interested in me than in any of your other patients.

THERAPIST: You would like to feel special.

MARTIN: You got it. You're right on target today. You must have seen your supervisor this week.

THERAPIST: I think your sarcasm may be your way of protecting yourself from letting me become important to you so that you do not risk being fooled and disappointed. It's easier to rely on coke even though it can be harmful to you than to count on me and expose yourself to being hurt again.

MARTIN: What if that's true?

THERAPIST: It's a dilemma for you. I think you want to trust me but it feels too dangerous. The more you feel that I understand you, the more you feel at risk and the more you have to protect yourself even at the price of hurting yourself.

MARTIN: I must admit that I can relate to what you're saying.

Borderline individuals often experience chronic feelings of narcissistic rage due to the severe and repeated assaults they experienced in early childhood. Their anger often overtakes them and also makes it particularly difficult for them to develop selfobject transferences. Magid (1984) suggests that when borderline patients ventilate their anger and mistrust of the world in general, and of the therapist in particular, it is important for the therapist to empathically relate to their feelings as understandable reactions to the emotional injuries they have experienced rather than to interpret their reactions as manifestations of pathological defenses such as splitting or projective identification. Otherwise, the therapist runs the risk of provoking more flagrant behavior, which in turn is viewed as evidence of a fixed borderline defensive structure.

MARTIN: The world is filled with imbeciles and incompetents who are rewarded with success while I have to work my ass off and get nothing for it! Do you know what my father had the nerve to say to me? He makes a ton of money and inherited even more and he has the nerve to tell me he's not going to loan me any more money, and that I should get a 9 to 5 job and stop fantasizing about what I'm going to do when I grow up. I would like to tear him limb from limb. By the way, I can't pay you this week. I'll give you a check at the end of the month. Is that all right? Well, if it's not all right, fuck you!

THERAPIST: I guess it's hard for you not to feel enraged that I'm going to be like all the other people in your life who don't deserve what they get and who don't give you what you deserve.

MARTIN: Why should you be different?

THERAPIST: I can understand why you feel that I will be like the rest based on your experience.

MARTIN: I don't always feel that way but you do stupid things sometimes.

THERAPIST: Tell me.

MARTIN: I just can't stand your being so understanding.

THERAPIST: What upsets you about that?

MARTIN: I don't know.

THERAPIST: Perhaps it makes it harder to be angry at and dismiss me and that makes you feel more vulnerable?

MARTIN: It also makes me realize how much time I spend being angry.

THERAPIST: You have had a lot of reasons to be angry.

Disruption and Repair of Selfobject Transferences

Once the selfobject transference becomes stable and operates smoothly, patients experience a sense of well-being and self-cohesion. Disruptions are inevitable, however, and commonly result from the therapist's lack of attunement to the patient's selfobject needs or failures in living up to the patients' expectations. Such disturbances result in a range of reactions, including narcissistic rage, disappointment, hurt, deidealization, depletion, and fragmentation. These disruptions must be repaired so that the selfobject transference can be restored. Repeated disruption–repair sequences provide the patient with experiences of "optimal frustration" that contribute to "transmuting internalizations" and the development of new self structures.

It is neither necessary or desirable to create disruptions in the selfobject transferences. They arise inevitably from the therapeutic process. First, the therapist is only human. He or she makes mistakes, or may fail to comprehend or respond empathically to all of the patient's selfobject needs. Second, the therapist is not perfect with respect to embodying all the characteristics that fit patients' idealizing needs. Third, the treatment has certain constraints: the therapist is not always available to the patient; sessions end; vacations and other types of temporary separations occur; interruptions for emergency telephone calls take place; and the therapist sometimes gets tired, sick, or has difficulty being emotionally present. Clearly, the atmosphere of the treatment and the therapists' general empathy and demeanor must be "good enough" to provide a stable back-drop in which temporary and nontraumatic disruptions occur.

The restoration of the therapist as a good selfobject results from the therapist's empathic exploration with the patient of how the disruptions occurred and of how these therapeutic lapses resemble earlier parental failures. *The therapist must try to understand and accept the validity of the patient's subjective experience, even if it is at variance with the therapist's perception of reality.* This is particularly important in work with borderline patients whose extreme reactions often seem to reflect gross distortions of the therapist's intentions, or to arise in reaction to what appear to be positive albeit threatening experiences in the treatment. A common impediment to this tactic is a therapist's fear that empathizing with a patient's seeming "distortions" or hypersensitivity will be experienced by the patient as approval of dysfunctional behavior. While the risk of this occurring exists, particularly with patients who show severe problems in reality testing, it is usually an unrealistic anxiety. There is a difference between trying to understand patients from their point of view and approving or condoning their behavior. Empathizing with patients does not prohibit therapists from sharing their own perceptions of the situation or their reasons for certain actions. The purpose of such explanations, however, is not to improve the patient's perceptions of reality, but rather to clarify where and how the disruption in the transference has taken place, in the service of repairing it and eventually understanding its connection to similar, more traumatic events in the patient's early life. When the selfobject bond is repaired, the patient's sense of well-being is restored and the treatment proceeds smoothly until the next such episode. These repeated disruption–restoration sequences both strengthen the selfobject connections and, over time, lead to transmuting internalizations that result in new and stronger self structures.

After Martin developed a somewhat more stable mirror transference with his therapist, he used his sessions to speak of his frustrated ambitions and his long-inhibited talents and interests. He often searched the therapist's face for signs of approval, and paid careful attention to the therapist's vocal intonations for indicators of her enthusiasm and interest. Simultaneously, Martin stopped using cocaine on a regular basis and began to devote more serious effort to both his acting career and to becoming financially self-supporting. Repeated disruptions of the transference occurred, however, and were always triggered either by Martin's perception of the therapist's insufficient attention to him or by unscheduled separations. While the early ruptures were set off by seemingly minor incidents and were accompanied by Martin's destructive acting-out, Martin became increasingly less upset by such events and was better able to maintain his sense of well-being despite their occurrence.

MARTIN: I know I'm ½ hour late but it's not my fault and I don't think I should have to pay you. The subway got stuck. I'm sick and tired of having to rush to get here. I don't know why you can't change my session time.

THERAPIST: You seem angry at me today.

MARTIN: I've been in an angry mood all week and I had a bad experience with coke that left me feeling terrible. It's all your fault.

THERAPIST: How so?

MARTIN: Do you think that I enjoyed watching you sneeze all through our last session? I don't know why you couldn't have taken something so that you could concentrate better. I'm not paying you to be sick during my session time.

THERAPIST: So you felt that I was not there for you even though I was physically present.

MARTIN: That's right!

THERAPIST: I can understand that you felt badly. How did that lead to your taking coke?

MARTIN: I wanted to feel better. You made me feel down. I thought I came in with good news last week about the acting coach who agreed to take me on as a student. Your response was to sneeze.

THERAPIST: You naturally wanted me to be enthusiastic and I let you down.

MARTIN: I thought you were more concerned about yourself than me.

THERAPIST: We've talked about how you've had a lot of experiences in which your parents have put your needs on the back-burner in favor of their own. Perhaps it's very important that I prove to you 100% that I'm there for you. If I slip a little, you feel frightened that you're going to be left with nothing.

MARTIN; Are you saying that I'm hypersensitive?

THERAPIST: I'm saying that you need a great deal of reassurance that people will be there for you and you are sensitive to any sign that they are going to fail you.

MARTIN: I felt very alone when I left here.

THERAPIST: You've had that feeling a lot in your life. You couldn't rely on others and you've had to turn to whatever you could to ease the pain. I guess that's where the coke comes in.

MARTIN: I still think you should take better care of yourself.

Understanding/Explaining Techniques

The two main technical interventions in self psychological treatment are understanding and explaining, two interrelated but conceptually different tools (Kohut, 1984; Ornstein & Ornstein, 1985; Wolf, 1988). Understanding refers to the therapist's empathic attunement to the patient as conveyed by statements, behavior, and nonverbal or even silent communication. It is different, however, from the therapist's attempts to explain or give meaning to what the patient displays or expresses in terms of its linkages to early childhood. What is explained in self psychological treatment differs from what is interpreted in treatments based on classical psychoanalytic theory or ego psychology. In self psychology the therapist focuses on the failures of the patients' early selfobject milieu and their impact on patients' personalities, rather than on instinctual conflicts and the defenses erected against them. Empathic explanations also contribute to the patient's feeling understood by the therapist. Understanding and explanation often occur together. Kohut emphasized, however, that a prolonged period of understanding without any attempts at explanation may be necessary with certain patients who have difficulty permitting the therapist to be separate from them in any way. These individuals experience the therapist's interpretations, however seemingly empathic, as unwanted intrusions.

With Martin the therapist was able to provide both understanding and explanation in some areas but not in others. For example, in the transference disruption described above, she not only attempted to show her understanding of both Martin's need for her to be enthusiastic and his response to what he felt was her lapse of attention, but she also attempted to explain his reaction in the light of early parental selfobject failures. For a long time in the treatment, however, when Martin looked to the therapist for actual mirroring, she was unable to explain the connection between Martin's dependence on external mirroring and the failures in his early life. He often ignored attempts at interpretation, and became more insistent on getting a desired response from the therapist, as the following example illustrates.

MARTIN: Yesterday I read for a part and I was fantastic. I'd like to bring it in and do it for you. What do you think?

THERAPIST: It seems important to you that I actually hear you do the part.

MARTIN: I want you to know how good I can be.

THERAPIST: I can understand your wanting that in light of how little appreciation and encouragement you have had in your life.

MARTIN: So, do you want to hear me read or not?

THERAPIST: I guess it is hard for you to feel sure that you are good if I don't validate your performance.

MARTIN: I don't know why you're giving me a hard time. All I want to do is read the part for you. I don't think you're really interested.

THERAPIST: I am interested.

MARTIN: Then just listen to me.

Using Mirroring Techniques

Many self psychologists take the position that psychoanalytic treatment should confine itself of understanding and explaining patients' selfobject needs rather than gratifying them. Some self psychological therapists (White and Weiner. 1986) believe that selectively providing an actual "mirroring" of the patient's needs for approval, admiration, or affective sharing, or responding to the patient in soothing and other need fulfilling ways, are important techniques particularly in the treatment of those individuals who have been severely deprived of selfobject experiences early in their lives. They argue that the distinction between what is or is not appropriate to psychoanalysis is arbitrary and has more to do with the lingering reliance on the traditional "abstinence" model than it does with what is therapeutically indicated. The willingness to use mirroring techniques does necessitate that the practitioner develop a set of criteria for when and with whom to provide mirroring. This involves a consideration of what will promote rather than inhibit the selfobject transference and the process of transmuting internalization. The use of mirroring techniques also does not preclude the use of explanation, and sometimes leads to patient responses that permit a further deepening of the patient's awareness of the links between his current and past needs.

With Martin a good deal of the treatment involved the therapist's provision not only of empathic understanding of Martin's mirroring needs as they appeared in the transference, but also of actual mirroring and attempts to repair the selfobject transference when her responses were felt to be inadequate. Sometimes when the therapist provided mirroring Martin became more accessible to explanations connecting his current behavior to the selfobject failures of his parents.

> MARTIN: I brought the part in to read to you.
> THERAPIST: Good. Let's hear it.
> MARTIN: I'm a little nervous.
> THERAPIST: What are you concerned about?
> MARTIN: I want you to like it but I'm afraid you'll be bored.
> THERAPIST: You're not sure you can trust my interest.
> MARTIN: Here goes. . . .
> THERAPIST: I enjoyed that.
> MARTIN: I thought you would. I'm a natural.
> THERAPIST: You should be pleased with yourself.
> MARTIN: Damn! I don't know why I'm feeling tearful.
> THERAPIST: What are you feeling?
> MARTIN: I wish I would have had someone like you when I was younger.
> THERAPIST: Well you should have had a lot more attention and encouragement than you did. Perhaps that's why you feel so hungry for it now and feel so terrible when you don't get as much as you'd like.

The Role of Confrontation

While Kohut argues that self psychologically informed interventions generally make confrontations unnecessary, in an unusual digression he reports a case in which he felt the need to use confrontation in order to draw attention to the patient's destructive acting-out. In this example

Kohut responded to a patient's unrepentant, angry account of his reckless driving and angry encounter with a police officer by telling the patient, "You are a complete idiot" (1984, p. 74). After the patient burst into friendly laughter, Kohut conveyed concern about certain potentially destructive aspects of the patient's behavior in numerous situations. He felt that this intervention led to a deeper understanding of what had precipitated the immediate incident, and of the dynamic roots of the patient's reactions in his early life. Kohut then states that "the self psychological orientation will not prevent the analyst from confronting the patient with the necessity of curbing his dangerous behavior, to control his 'acting-out'" (1984, p. 75). It is curious that Kohut, however, never indicates why he chose to confront the patient rather than address his reaction somewhat differently, does not elaborate on the criteria to be used for making such an intervention, and omits discussing whether he thought it was an optimal intervention or a countertransferential response that nevertheless worked in this instance.

It is an open question whether it is always possible to contain some borderline patients' impulsiveness and tendencies toward destructive behavior through empathic understanding and responsiveness alone. More active interventions may be necessary with some borderline patients in order to safeguard the treatment, and the patient's life. Within an empathic framework it is possible to use limits and structure and to show concern about the patient's behavior, but these interventions have not been well-described from a self psychological perspective. The therapist's ability to integrate "empathic confrontations" and the use of external structure into a self psychological treatment, as is shown in the example below, may enable such treatment to be successful with the more impulse-ridden borderline individuals.

The therapist's unanticipated absence for several weeks after one year of treatment resulted in a resurgence of Martin's cocaine abuse. Upon her return, the therapist persistently tried to repair the disruption in the transference, but Martin was inconsolable. Despite his coming to sessions, her attempts to empathize with his pain and anger were to no avail. He had felt totally abandoned and helpless when the therapist was away. While he knew how to contact her through her answering machine, he did not know exactly where she was at any given time. Concerned about the severity of the cocaine abuse and Martin's deteriorating condition, the therapist felt she needed to address this directly in the treatment.

MARTIN: I'm here but I have nothing to say.

THERAPIST: I know you feel that I have caused you great pain, and are having trouble forgiving me and letting me have another chance, but there's something I need to say to you.

MARTIN: What?

THERAPIST: I'm very concerned about you. I can't just sit by and watch you destroy yourself with drugs.

MARTIN: I don't want to talk about it. It's the only thing that relieves me.

THERAPIST: I don't want to cause you more pain but I also do not want you to wind up dead.

MARTIN: I can handle it.

THERAPIST: It's not a sign of your weakness that you can't handle it. Drugs take on a life of their own.

MARTIN: I don't want to talk about it.

THERAPIST: Whatever has happened to make you want to destroy yourself is something we may not be able to work out right now, but your survival and well-being are important. I can't make you stop abusing coke but I really want you to take action.

MARTIN: What do you want me to do?

THERAPIST: Have you considered going to a drug program?

MARTIN: Are you kidding?

THERAPIST: I'm quite serious. It is very hard to stop on your own. What you're doing isn't working.

MARTIN: You're some therapist. You go away and leave me alone and then you want to push me off on a stupid drug program. I'm going to walk out of here.

THERAPIST: I hope you won't do that. I know you are still in a rage at me and feel I don't care about you, but I have to get through to you about the importance of your caring enough about yourself to take care of the drugs now. I want you to think about it and come up with a plan.

Martin got up and, slamming the door, left the office. He called the therapist the same evening and apologized. He said he would think about what she said. He did want to get off drugs. He was going to try to stop and if he was not successful, he would go to Narcotics Anonymous.

Countertransference Issues

There are a variety of potential stresses on the self psychological therapist that stem from: (1) the therapist's own archaic grandiosity, omnipotence, and needs for mirroring and idealization — for example, and the defenses erected against them that may be stimulated by the necessary regression that occurs in the therapist that enables empathic understanding; (2) the intensity of the patient's archaic selfobject needs and the verbal and emotional assaults on the therapist, or the sometimes severe regressions or acting-out that occurs when these are frustrated or misunderstood; (3) a patient's frustration of the therapist's "normal" need to be recognized as a distinct person and appreciated, (4) the vulnerability of the therapist because of a difficult or nonrewarding personal or professional life; (5) the demands on the therapist to understand how his or her own reactions have contributed to disruptions of the selfobject transference; (6) the process of trying to be a good selfobject to patients while not having had good selfobject experiences in one's own life or personal psychotherapy; (7) needs for status and feelings of competence; and (8) the lack of professional support for a non-traditional treatment approach that can be turbulent and demanding and which may go against some of their own training.

ADLER AND BUIE'S MIXED MODEL OF PSYCHOTHERAPY

In contrast to Brandchaft and Stolorow, Gerald Adler (1985) and Adler and Daniel Buie (1982) see borderline pathology as a stable and distinctive disorder that is characterized by the individual's lack of sustaining introjects. Consequently, they believe that treatment must encompass some additional features beyond those that self psychology advocates. They have put forth a mixed approach that draws on psychoanalytic ego psychology, object-relations theory, and self psychology.

Treatment Goals and Framework

The goal of therapy is to help borderline individuals, who lack the ability to evoke positive, sustaining images of others in their absence or when frustrated by them, to develop the capacity for evocative memory. Since Adler and Buie argue that it is the absence of positive introjects rather than the characteristic splitting that Kernberg emphasizes that leads to the borderline patient's overwhelming sense of aloneness and unmodulated rage, they seek to foster new internalizations rather than to confront and interpret pathological defenses. Drawing on Winnicott's view that therapy, like "good-enough mothering," should provide a relationship of safety, security, and trust, Adler and Buie emphasize the importance of a therapeutic "holding environment," especially in the beginning phase and during the patient's stormy periods throughout the treatment. Such an atmosphere is essential to help patients contain their anxiety, to enable them to internalize the therapist as a positive introject, and to develop the capacity for evocative memory. This acquisition will permit patients to overcome their terrible, chronic states of aloneness, panic, rage, and emptiness that occur when they are separated from those upon whom they depend for sustenance, as well as their fears of abandonment, which keep them from developing close attachments. Likewise, the pathological defenses and destructive patterns that they have used to cope with their turbulent inner experiences will be replaced by more adaptive behavior, and they will develop greater psychological stability, self-sufficiency, and self-worth.

The framework of the treatment generally calls for face-to-face psychotherapy two to five times a week. In the beginning of the treatment, when borderline patients tend to show more impulsive and destructive behavior, limits need to be established to protect the patient. Such measures, however, are one small part of the establishment of a holding environment that is accessible and sustaining enough for the patient's experience of aloneness to be kept within tolerable bounds. The specific elements that make up the proper therapeutic structure and ambience will vary with the needs of the patient. In many instances the therapist will need to be available to the patient outside of regular session times. Brief telephone calls, extra appointments, and the use of transitional objects such as vacation addresses and postcards may be necessary to help patients contain their feelings and impulses and maintain their positive connection to the therapist during periods of separation, however seemingly brief. In some instances the devastating impact of longer separations — over summer vacations, for example — may actually require some patients to be hospitalized.

The Nature of the Therapeutic Relationship

The Therapist as a Selfobject

Because of their severe deficits, borderline individuals require actual selfobject functioning by the therapist in addition to empathic understanding and interpretation. At the beginning of their treatment they are not really capable of a therapeutic alliance or a collaborative partnership with the therapist. Their need for fusion or merger and fears of abandonment are too great. Likewise, their feelings of aloneness are easily stimulated and often intolerable. The therapist must actively find ways of helping them to bear their feelings as well as sustain them sufficiently for them to develop a selfobject transference. When such a transference occurs and deepens, the patient's regression can be quite tumultuous. The therapist may need to be available by

left treatment and led a chaotic life until going back to college in her senior year. There she saw a supportive and reality oriented woman social worker once a week who also lived in Nancy's dormitory and was involved in numerous campus activities. Nancy was able to make contact with her frequently during the week by ascertaining the therapist's schedule and arranging for "accidental" encounters in which they would exchange nods or verbal greetings. Their relationship was not particularly intense and this unusual arrangement seemed to help assuage Nancy's abandonment fears, separation anxiety, and the panic that was present in the first treatment.

The social worker who had helped Nancy get through school, a major achievement in itself, did not attempt to deal with her more severe and longstanding personality difficulties. When she began her third treatment with another woman therapist on a twice a week basis, Nancy formed an intense but constantly shifting relationship with her. She seemed to have little ability to "take the therapist with her," so to speak, when Nancy would leave the sessions. She became anxious and fearful, and dealt with this in several ways: she made suicide threats as she was closing the door to the office; she would take extra time to write a check to pay for the session or would refuse to leave; she would try to reconnect with her by calling, sometimes within minutes of leaving the session, from a nearby telephone booth to ask if the therapist liked her; she asked for personal information to help her visualize where the therapist was and what she was doing when Nancy was not with her; and she asked to tape record parts of sessions so that she could hear the therapist's voice. If Nancy was not able to make the desired positive contact with the therapist she became more desperate and enraged, and often left messages that she was quitting treatment or about to kill herself. If the therapist was not totally attuned to Nancy's often confusing communications in the sessions themselves, she would shift from a seemingly positive way of relating to a verbal attack on the therapist's character and personality traits. Yet, if the therapist was empathic, Nancy became distrustful and accusatory.

Despite the overtly aggressive and controlling aspects of Nancy's behavior, the therapist understood Nancy's problems as stemming from an absence of internal positive introjects and structures for self-soothing. These core deficits led to severe panic states, unmodulated rage reactions, and desperate attempts to make herself feel better by maintaining contact with the therapist at any cost. Even highly charged negative interactions, in which she suffered and felt victimized, felt better than having no contact. Commenting on or interpreting Nancy's angry and controlling behavior only escalated her sense of aloneness and anger. Empathizing with her desperation and trying to sensitively relate to the stimuli that set Nancy off were more soothing temporarily, but did not hold her sufficiently. Supplementing this more empathic stance, the therapist explained Nancy's problem to her in ways she could assimilate, and while adhering to the treatment structure, tried to ease the separation when she left the sessions as shown in the following brief vignettes.

NANCY: Why do I have to leave the session? It's not fair that you get to decide when my time is up.

THERAPIST: I do have another patient waiting.

NANCY: I'm not important to you. It doesn't matter how upset I feel. Time's up. Dismissed!

THERAPIST: I know it doesn't feel good to have to leave when you're not ready. You feel very alone and cut-off from me. You begin to trust me when you're here and then when you leave it is hard for you to continue to feel that I care and am there for you.

NANCY: Can't I stay longer? I have so much to talk about.

THERAPIST: Perhaps you could write your thoughts and feelings down during the week and we'll talk about them next time?

NANCY: That's a good idea. I can think of your reactions when I'm writing. I'll leave but I have to write out your check. You want to get paid don't you? I forgot to do it before I got here.

THERAPIST: I know you want to stay and are upset that you have to leave but I would prefer that you finish this up in the waiting room. You can stay there for a little while if you like.

NANCY: Okay. Okay. I know I'm being difficult.

THERAPIST: I think it's hard for you to get close and then have to separate. What might help you?

NANCY: I need a 5 minute warning before the end of the session.

THERAPIST: We can try that.

Limit-Setting, Confrontation, and Interpretation

In addition to helping patients to control impulses that are harmful to themselves and others, the therapist's setting of limits "can be a new experience for the patient with a person who appropriately cares and protects" (Adler, 1985, p. 212). This is particularly important with patients who have backgrounds of deprivation and neglect. The therapist's passivity in the face of a patient's out of control or otherwise destructive behavior can signal a repetition of the inadequacies of their early caretakers. At the same time, setting limits also interferes with the autonomy of patients, who may feel that the therapist is trying to control them. This issue is confounded by the fact that the therapist may set limits, in part, because he or she is unable to tolerate the patient's behavior. Such an intervention is legitimate as a statement of who the therapist is but also risks exposing the therapist's limitations or incapacities. On the other hand, some therapists may deny the danger related to the patient's behavior. There are tradeoffs therapeutically between protection and the support of autonomy as well as between omnipotence and anxiety.

Optimally, limits should be established thoughtfully rather than as a consequence of the therapist's anger or frustrations. Sometimes the failure to set appropriate limits in a timely way makes the therapist more vulnerable to counteraggressive attacks on the patient when the latter's behavior exceeds the therapist's tolerance.

The therapist clarifies, confronts, and interprets patients' feelings and behavior in order to help them understand their inner experience and reactions, to enable them to use the therapy to lessen maladaptive defenses, to block destructive acting out, and to enable them to deal with reality. These techniques, however, need to be used carefully and as part of the therapist's efforts to help the patient sustain a positive holding relationship, which is the *sine qua non* of this treatment model.

According to Adler (1985, pp. 121–122), the main purpose of confrontation, which focuses patients' attention on inner experiences or perceptions of outer reality of which they are conscious or about which they are to be made conscious, is to overcome their resistances to such recognition. Confrontation should be used sparingly to counter maladaptive defenses and the destructive behavior resulting from them, and in urgent situations where patients are misperceiving reality or endangering themselves. Confrontation should not be used when it increases the stress patients are already experiencing due to a disturbing reality situation, breaks down needed defenses, overstimulates the patient's wish for closeness or rage, or points out narcissistic entitlement and unrealistic wishes.

Because of some of the more flagrant and potentially self-destructive behavior Nancy engaged in, it was necessary for the therapist to set limits and use confrontation and interpretation selectively.

NANCY: I'm calling from the subway. I'm waiting for a train. I forgot to tell you that my boss told me I was the best assistant he's ever had. What do you think of that?

THERAPIST: I think you deserve his praise but I can't really talk now.

NANCY: I have to ask you something. I need your advice.

THERAPIST: This is really not a good time for me to talk. I really need to hang up now.

NANCY: You should schedule more time between patients. I've got to go anyway. My train is coming.

NANCY: If you never see me again, it's because I killed myself.

THERAPIST: Do you really mean that or are you angry about having to leave the session?

NANCY: You decide.

THERAPIST: I think you're angry about having to leave the session. You told me today that you were beginning to trust me more. Now you have to leave and that is making you feel that I'm abandoning you.

NANCY: So what are you going to do?

THERAPIST: I will be here to see you during our sessions and you know you can call me if you need to but now I must see another patient.

THERAPIST: Your mother called me today to say that you had locked yourself in your room last night and she was frantic that you were going to hurt yourself until she convinced you to let her in.

NANCY: I was furious that she called you.

THERAPIST: Perhaps you were angry at me for taking her call?

NANCY: A little, but you told me in the beginning that you would talk to her if she became concerned about me.

THERAPIST: It sounds like you knew she would call me. What were you feeling that made you lock yourself in your room?

NANCY: I just felt bad and I promised that I wouldn't call you after 10 P.M.

THERAPIST: I guess you felt that if I really cared about you I would let you call whenever you needed to.

NANCY: When you're not there I get desperate and feel suicidal.

THERAPIST: Your parents became frightened when you locked yourself in your room. I know you felt bad but when you do things like that they get scared. If you really want to hurt yourself I have to take your threats seriously.

NANCY: I mean it at the moment.

THERAPIST: How do I know that you won't do something about it?

NANCY: I want you to worry.

THERAPIST: I think we have to find another way for you to get the reassurance you need that I care about you and still am here without you're having to threaten to hurt yourself. I'm willing to do what I can to be there for you, but I also need you to promise that you will let me know if you really don't think you can control yourself, and that you will not use suicide threats as a way of getting me to be concerned.

NANCY: I don't know if I can promise that.

THERAPIST: What do you think might help you to hold onto good feelings about me and yourself when you feel upset so that you can promise?

NANCY: I don't know.

THERAPIST: What is it like for you when you are home alone?

NANCY: It's different at different times. Sometimes I feel like I don't have anyone to love except you and I feel I have to talk to you.

THERAPIST You said there were other feelings too.

NANCY: My parents upset me and I feel like a bad person. I have to get rid of the feeling.

THERAPIST: I don't mind talking to you briefly if that helps, but sometimes I'm not available. You may get more desperate and angry if you can't reach me or if I'm busy. You can leave a message and I'll call you back. Even if I can't always be there when you need me, it doesn't mean that I don't care.

NANCY: I don't like to wait.

THERAPIST: Is there something else that would help?

NANCY: Sometimes I would like to have something in your handwriting or a picture or something. That's it. Can I take your picture? I can look at it and keep it with me. Maybe you could autograph it. I'll have my own shrink at all times.

THERAPIST: There's no harm in trying if you think it will help.

NANCY: I feel better just thinking about doing it. See you next week.

NANCY: I really hate you.

THERAPIST: What have I done?

NANCY: It's what you don't do. All you do is sit there and listen and talk.

THERAPIST: What would you like?

NANCY: Fuck off! You don't care about me.

THERAPIST: I think you are getting scared about feeling that I do care. You are feeling vulnerable and by being angry you are pushing me away, but then when you push me away you feel abandoned and alone. It's a bind for you.

NANCY: So when are you going on vacation?

THERAPIST: Why do you ask that?

NANCY: You haven't gone away since I've known you. I figure you must be getting ready for a vacation.

THERAPIST: As a matter of fact, I will be away for a week next month. I was going to tell you that today.

NANCY: Where are you going?

THERAPIST: Is it important for you to know?

NANCY: You're probably afraid I'll track you down and call you. I won't. It would just help me to know where you are — the city or country — not where you're staying necessarily.

THERAPIST: I'm going to San Francisco.

NANCY: That's far. Will you send me a postcard? Then I'll know you are thinking about me.

THERAPIST: I can do that but I may get back before the postcard arrives given the United States mail.

NANCY: That's okay so long as I know you're sending it.

Optimal Disillusionment

The second phase of treatment is characterized by the use of Kohut's disruption–restoration sequence in a process of optimal disillusionment of the holding–soothing aspects of the therapist's selfobject functions. Reality constraints and the therapist's humaneness result in discrepancies between patients' wishes for an idealized holding introject who is always there for them and the therapist's ability to deliver. If the disappointments in the therapist are not too traumatic — that is, they do not lead to severe regressions, overwhelming rage and aloneness, or irreparable disruptions of the treatment — the unrealistic idealizations of the therapist can be worked through and relinquished. "Ultimately the therapist as holding selfobject is accepted as he realistically is: an interested, caring person who, in the context of a professional relationship, does all that he appropriately can to help the patient resolve conflicts and achieve mature capacities" (Adler, 1985, p. 60). Thus, optimal disillusionment leads to transmuting internalizations.

This process requires that the therapist understands the nature of the patient's disappointments and, through clarification and interpretation, connects them to their earlier roots in the patient's life. Confrontations concerning the unrealistic quality of the patient's wishes for an idealized holding object or extreme reactions when disappointed or frustrated should not be made as these would likely intensify the disruptions. These episodes of disillusionment often result in a painful grief process in which patients fully recognize their past deprivations and relinquish their impossible yearnings along with the acquisition of needed holding introjects.

Since many borderline patients also show severe narcissistic difficulties and problems related to grandiosity and feelings of worthlessness, treatment of the narcissistic sector of borderline pathology can be woven into the general treatment through the disruption and repair of selfobject transferences following Kohut. Adler cautions, however, that this work requires that patients have established sufficiently stable holding introjects as a result of the treatment of their primary pathology.

The following vignette from a later phase in Nancy's treatment illustrates the disruption–restoration sequence.

NANCY: I'm feeling suicidal. I really am.

THERAPIST: When did you start feeling this way?

NANCY: Last week. I haven't wanted to go to work all week. I stayed home sick for a few days.

THERAPIST: Perhaps you are reacting to my going away for a month?

NANCY: I don't understand you. You just announce that you're going to be on vacation for a month and I'm supposed to close off all my needs and feelings while you have a good time. You try to get me to feel that you care and then you make a unilateral decision that does not take me into account at all. What do you want me to feel? You think because I'm doing better that I don't need you any more.

THERAPIST: I guess it makes you feel helpless and that you don't matter.

NANCY: I don't want to even talk to you. I don't know why I bother coming to see you. I'm going to stop if I don't kill myself first.

THERAPIST: Is it that you're fearful of what will happen when I'm away or that you just feel terribly left out and abandoned?

NANCY: Both. Last time you went away I panicked one night. I didn't know how to reach you. I know I could have called your answering machine but I didn't know when you would get your messages. It was as if you didn't exist. I was totally alone. If I died you wouldn't even know.

THERAPIST: That was a terrible state to be in.

NANCY: Even your picture didn't help. The only thing that helped was writing you a letter to the vacation address you gave me.

THERAPIST: I remember. So you are worried that you will feel that way again and angry at me for not considering that.

NANCY: I have been doing better so I guess you think I can get along without you.

THERAPIST: You have been doing better but I don't know why you think I won't be available to you in the ways I have been previously during vacation.

NANCY: You haven't taken a month off before.

THERAPIST: It feels like too long to hold out. It reminds me of the times when you were a child and your parents would leave you with your aunt and not call because they thought you were taken care of.

NANCY: I couldn't understand that they thought she was a substitute.

THERAPIST: What's more painful for you is that they weren't there for you when they were home. Then when they left you had nothing to hold on to. Do you feel that way with me?

NANCY: No. Not any more. You have been there and sometimes I find myself talking to myself the way you would talk to me. Is that bad?

THERAPIST: I think it's good that you can do that for yourself.

NANCY: When you're away I find myself paying special attention to the news about the city you're in and the weather and things like that. I try to visualize what you are doing. Where are you going this time?

THERAPIST: Easthampton.

NANCY: Again? You're in a rut.

Providing a Variety of Selfobject Functions

In the later phases of treatment, when the patient's selfobject transference is established more securely, the therapist functions as a selfobject in a variety of ways that provide the basis for positive identifications and internalizations. Ego and superego development occurs. Patients evolve a self-holding capacity that allows them to care about their own well-being, the ability to love themselves and others, trust and security in their competence, prideful enjoyment of their abilities, self-esteem, and guiding standards and values, with the internal authority to promote them.

NANCY: I'm furious at my boss. I've been working late every night to do some new lay-outs and he didn't even look at them before he went away. Maybe they aren't any good?

THERAPIST: I can understand your disappointment and anger that he didn't look at them but you seem to be down on yourself. Your work is of value whether or not he looks at it.

NANCY: I brought the drawings in. I want to know what you think of them.

THERAPIST: You know I'm not an expert in this area.

NANCY: I just want you to see them.

THERAPIST: I'll be glad to look at them, but I also think it's important that you hold on to your sense of your own talent even if your boss is not available.

NANCY: So what do you think?

THERAPIST: They look dynamic and colorful.

NANCY: I'm glad you picked up on the color. I thought I would experiment a little.

THERAPIST: No one in your family was interested in encouraging your abilities, or was there to comfort you when you ran into difficulty.

NANCY: I don't want to talk about that.I don't want to have to analyze everything. It makes me sad.

THERAPIST: It is sad and it helps to explain how easily you get upset when someone isn't there for you.

Countertransference Issues

Countertransference reactions in the therapist that can obstruct the treatment are commonly stimulated by the borderline patient's devaluing attitudes and behavior. This characteristic tendency arises because of patients' rage, fears of abandonment, and their the need to protect against wishes for nurture, envy, projected anger, and low self-esteem. Therapists often react to devaluation with: (1) feelings of helplessness and hopelessness about the patient's ability to get better; (2) worthlessness and depression regarding their therapeutic abilities; (3) guilt and shame for not being able to rescue the patient or live up to the patient's expectations of their therapist's omnipotence; (4) envy of the patient's demands for unconditional care and nurture; and (5) regression leading to excessive self doubt about the value of therapy and their career choice. Unless their reactions are understood and resolved, therapists are likely to cope in ways that are countertherapeutic. They may withdraw from the patient in order to protect themselves, attempt to prove their omnipotence and love by extreme acts of dedication, retaliate through inappropriate confrontations and interpretations of the patient's aggressive behavior, or deny the patient's hostility by interpreting anger as masking love.

CONCLUSION

The three deficit-based treatment models that this chapter has described and illustrated reflect basic similarities and some important differences such as their treatment goals and framework, views of the nature of the therapeutic relationship, main techniques and principal features, and outlook on countertransference. Whether emphasizing ego building, the strengthening of the self, or the development of sustaining introjects, each aims at ameliorating early defects through enabling patients to develop new internalizations. All recommend a stable yet flexible and individualized treatment structure. Adler and Buie alone address the need for setting limits on potentially destructive behavior. Both Kohut's self psychological approach and Adler and Buie's mixed model stress the provision of an attuned or "good-enough holding environment" in which the therapist's empathic understanding of the patient's subjective experience is important. The Blancks's emphasis on the therapist's attention to the patient's subphase needs reflects an appreciation of the role of the real relationship, but they remain more "objective" and experience-distant in their interventions. The self psychologists are unique in their stress on the intersubjective nature of the patient–therapist interaction.

All the theorists recognize that borderline patients form different types of relationships or transferences in treatment than those described by traditional psychoanalysis. These require special understanding and responses. While taking somewhat different positions on the provision of emotionally corrective experiences, these models share the view that the experiential and reparative aspects of the treatment are as important as its content. Each model redefines the nature and content of interpretation differently from its traditional meaning and cautiously uses confrontation, with the self psychological group employing this technique the least. All models provide some type of support. Self psychology is the least normative of the models with respect to what is desirable behavior, and emphasizes the creativity and uniqueness of the self. Each approach recognizes the patient's impact on the therapist in stimulating countertransference reactions but focuses more on the therapist's personal vulnerability to potentially harmful attitudes and responses. This is particularly true of the self psychological approach which sees most disruptions in the treatment as stemming from unattuned therapeutic responses.

8

Towards an Integrative
Clinical Perspective

Each of the treatment models described in Chapters 6 and 7 is based on different conceptions of the nature and development of borderline disorders. While showing some common features, the various conflict- and deficit-based approaches reflect diametrically opposed views of the goals and framework of treatment, the nature of the therapeutic relationship, the types of interventions to be used, and the meaning of countertransference. Several important questions arise in considering these diverse treatment models. What are the strengths and weaknesses of each approach? Is there one ideal treatment for all patients, or an optimal fit between a treatment model and a particular patient at a given time? Can the conflict and deficit models be reconciled? Do borderline individuals show a range of developmental pathology that necessitates an individualized and flexible treatment approach? How does the clinician decide what to do with whom? In considering these questions this chapter first will critique the various models and then will discuss the elements of an integrative clinical perspective in the treatment of borderline disorders.

CRITIQUE OF MAJOR TREATMENT MODELS

Kernberg's Model

Kernberg's approach is powerful in helping borderline individuals to contain their destructive and self-defeating behavior, and in helping them to identify their pathological defenses and internalized self- and object-representations. It offers the clearest guidelines to the interventive process, but it is a rigid and inflexible model. The Kernbergian therapist is neutral, abstinent, and confident in his or her view of what is wrong with the patient and what constitutes mature, realistic behavior. He or she does not have to struggle with how and when to use the therapeutic relationship differentially to foster the patient's growth, to selectively meet the patient's needs, or to support the patient's moves toward greater autonomy. In setting an unwavering treatment structure and clear limits on acting-out and other types of seemingly undesirable intrusions on the therapy, therapists who follow this approach need not extend themselves beyond traditionally prescribed bounds and contractual arrangements. From the beginning of treatment the therapist is able to authoritatively clarify, confront, and interpret patients' primitive defenses that center on the splitting off of aggression, pathological self- and object-representations, destructive attitudes and behavior, and angry or dismissive reactions to therapist interventions. When feeling attacked, devalued, or helpless the therapist looks to what the patient is inducing in him or her and uses these reactions as diagnostic of the patient's projected and split-off inner states.

This model is problematic in numerous ways, even if one accepts its basic assumption that borderline disorders reflect problems with aggression resulting in pathological defenses and internalized object relations. It is questionable whether therapeutic change can be achieved entirely through such an unrelenting assault on this pathology in the absence of a more directly supportive and empathic relationship that attempts to foster new internalizations. While Kernberg's argument that the borderline patient's aggression interferes with the development of the therapeutic alliance may be true in many instances, often this anger may be a justifiable reaction to the therapist's insensitivity or the result of fear. Further, it is likely that the extensive use of confrontation early in the treatment and during times of acute distress will escalate rather than diffuse the patient's anger. Along with therapeutic neutrality, confrontation will be too readily experienced by many patients as attacking, withholding, critical, and a replay of past traumatic relationships that warrant aggressive or mistrustful responses. Moreover, the therapist's expert or know-it-all attitude about what is going on with patients and what is best for them communicates that what they think and feel is not valid. While sometimes confrontation can be felt as caring, it is rarely, if ever experienced as empathic, even when based on a correct "objective" view of a patient's contradictory or self-defeating attitudes or behavior. While it is conceivable that this contradiction in the ways that empathy and confrontation are experienced by patients can be overcome by carefully framed comments, the style of Kernberg's interventions are harsh. Borderline patients need to be shown that their worst fantasies are not true. Lastly, the rigid or mechanical use of limits and contracts with patients creates demands on them to be healthier than they are. If they were able to control their impulses easily, they would not be in such desperate straits. It also justifies therapist noninvolvement and insensitivity.

Kernberg's clarity about the nature of borderline pathology and his precise treatment recommendations do not fit all those individuals in the borderline spectra described by others. The differences in perspectives on borderline pathology reflect more than the fact that clinicians variously interpret similar clinical features (for example, seeing idealization as a defense rather than as a search for an archaic selfobject). There are a vast number of patients who share the borderline diagnosis who do not seem to show the stable defensive structure revolving around splitting of all "good" and all "bad" self- and object-representations. Their ego and self structures have not consolidated and they show a variety of deficits that need to be addressed. In contrast, Kernberg assumes that ego functions and a stable, cohesive identity will develop once patients overcome splitting.

Kernberg's model does not consider whether there are those individuals who need more direct help in building ego, internalizing new self- and object-representations, or strengthening the self. Similarly, he omits consideration of whether the treatment goals, framework, and technical interventions need to be more flexible and individualized with such patients. His emphasis on limit-setting and external structure helps to contain destructive impulses but does not ameliorate feelings of desperation and aloneness, nor do they foster the development of self-soothing capacities. His minimization of the impact of actual traumatic events in early childhood, such as parental neglect, physical and sexual abuse, serious problems in attunement, and illness and death, lends itself to empathic failures by the therapist.

The potential benefit of using the therapeutic relationship as a reparative experience is grossly underestimated, if not depreciated by Kernberg. Some patients need more from the treatment than they can get from insight into their maladaptive patterns. Many cannot tolerate the interventions that Kernberg proposes in either his expressive or supportive psychotherapy. They need help in developing trustworthy human relationships, in differentiating and separating themselves from others, in identifying and verbalizing their inner experience, and in getting validation for their rights and feelings. They need to feel safe before they can reexperience and work through the emotional pain and narcissistic injuries of the past to any degree.

Finally, while the concept of induced countertransference is important in work with many disturbed patients, Kernberg applies it too globally. His tendency to confront and interpret what the patient is "putting into" the therapist through the defense of projective identification and angry or defensive reactions to therapeutic interventions risks giving therapists a rationale for self-serving, counteraggressive attacks on patients whose behavior is provocative and annoying, as well as for other types of countertransference acting-out (Reiser & Levenson, 1984). The therapist's willingness to scrutinize his or her internal attitudes and feelings and to consider how he or she has contributed to the patient's regressive, turbulent, or even destructive reactions can be an important experience in human relations.

Masterson's Model

This approach seems especially suited to those borderline individuals whose main difficulties are related to their clinging and dependent behavior on the one hand, and their fears of autonomy and independence on the other. As in Kernberg's model, stability and firmness in the treatment framework and clear guidelines for technical interventions are helpful in enabling patients to control and understand their destructive or self-defeating behavior. Masterson, however, seems to assume that verbal interventions are generally sufficient to help patients contain their impulses, and does not focus on the use of limits or external structure except in those instances where hospitalization may be necessary.

Masterson's use of confrontation of what are considered to be regressive yearnings and defenses early in treatment can be helpful in altering the overt behavior of those patients who can tolerate this approach. For those many other patients who may need a period of acceptance of their dependent needs, this technique risks interfering with rather than building a therapeutic alliance and cuts off what may be a necessary stage in the treatment.

In emphasizing the one major dynamic of abandonment depression and the split rewarding and withdrawing part object-relations units, this approach is very specific but also narrow in its scope. Many borderline patients do not present with the organized set of defenses, the distinct internalized object-relations split, or the family patterns that Masterson and Rinsley describe. Their object-relations pathology is more pervasive or diffuse and their family backgrounds are more traumatic and varied. Abuse and neglect are frequent, in addition to the rewarding of regressive behavior and the punishment of individuation through the withdrawal of love. Ego functions are much more disturbed and self-esteem is poor.

In stressing both extensive confrontation and empathy, Masterson minimizes the problems in using two diametrically opposite techniques. By advocating the therapist's active encouragement and support of patients' appropriate strivings for autonomy, however, he does show some regard for the reparative aspects of the treatment relationship and corrects for Kernberg's too rigid emphasis on the therapist's technical neutrality and abstinence. Nevertheless, by deliberately utilizing the combination of confrontation of regressive (bad) behavior and positive acknowledgment and enthusiasm for independent (good) strivings, the therapist takes a judgmental, normative, and manipulative stance. The model seems to view autonomy as the *sine qua non* of mental health and does not sufficiently address other important capacities, such as the capacity for mutuality and mature dependence. The therapist is allowed to be real and to support the patient but only in the area of the patient's individuation.

Gertrude and Rubin Blancks's Model

The Blancks's treatment model is well-suited to those borderline patients whose ego deficits seem to require a more directly supportive approach. These patients have difficulty tolerating confrontation and generally do not show a rigid defensive structure. This model is more flexible in its framework and interventions than both Kernberg's and Masterson's approaches. Like Masterson, the Blancks focus mainly on separation–individuation issues but address numerous subphase difficulties rather than one core problem. In advocating a variety of ego building techniques and real object experiences in which there is measured gratification of patients' needs, this model is directly supportive. In minimizing confrontation, particularly in the earlier stages of treatment, it is relatively accepting and nonassaultive of patients' defenses. Since the therapy is not focused primarily on the control of behavior through the establishment of firm limits, external structure, and the use of confrontation, it may not be as effective as other models with highly impulse-ridden and self-destructive patients.

The Blancks's model is more sensitive to understanding and responding to patients' needs as the patient experiences them than are Kernberg's and Masterson's approaches. The therapist's provision of real object experiences and measured gratification reflects an emphasis on the experiential and reparative aspects of the treatment process. At the same time, the Blancks show a certain reticence or ambivalence about the role of gratification in psychotherapy since they indicate that it is only permissible for therapists to meet some of the needs of very disturbed patients. Their interventions are more conservative in practice than in principle. Their expectations that patients be autonomous, mature, and reality oriented reflect their normative value system. While discussing the importance of self-esteem, their approach does not really focus on improving self-feelings.

This model requires more creativity and experimentation in regard to the therapists' use of themselves in the treatment process than do Kernberg's and Masterson's approaches. Unfortunately, the criteria for when and how to provide real object experiences and measured gratification are not well spelled out. Consequently, therapists using this model must struggle to find optimal ways of intervening in each case. This places special demands on therapists to be uniquely responsive to patients and to be cautious and self-scrutinizing with respect to meeting the patient's needs rather than their own.

Kohut's Self Psychological Model

Kohut's self psychological approach and Kernberg's object-relations model are diametrically opposed in many respects. For instance, in self psychological treatment a human and empathic ambience replaces limits and firmness; experience-near-empathy takes precedence over therapeutic neutrality; selfobject transferences are allowed to unfold rather than be confronted and interpreted; empathic understanding and explanation of early failures in attunement, rather than confrontation and interpretation of aggression and defenses are the main techniques; the experiential and reparative nature of the treatment relationship is more important than the content of interventions; the patient's subjective feelings and experiences take priority over the therapist's objective or expert observations; patients' uniqueness, lifelong selfobject needs, and efforts at self expression rather than their conformity and autonomy are valued; disruptions in the treatment are the responsibility of the therapist rather than attributed to the patient's pathology; and in some instances, gratification supersedes abstinence.

According to Brandchaft and Stolorow (1984a, 1984b) and White and Weiner (1986), there are no limitations to the use of this model with borderline patients. The powerful impact of empathic attunement will "hold" patients even amidst inevitable and stormy disruptions and enable them to develop the stable selfobject transferences necessary for the approach to be successful. There are no additional parameters or alterations in technique with those borderline patients who are highly impulse-ridden, need to ward off closeness to preserve a sense of self, show serious ego as well as self deficits, or who seem dominated by "bad" internal objects. It is not clear from reading their cases whether Brandchaft and Stolorow have worked extensively with borderline patients who show these more flagrant difficulties.

The "pure" self psychological approach is best suited to those borderline individuals who show significant self pathology that can be contained sufficiently by empathic attunement so that their lives or the lives of others are not endangered by their destructive or self-defeating behavior, and who are not so emotionally endangered by a selfobject transference that they withdraw or fragment as a reaction to certain types of empathy. With other borderline patients treatment based on self psychological principles requires some expansion and variation in order to be useful. For example, taking a more active and concerned stance that possibly includes limit-setting may be necessary when patients are engaging in potentially harmful behavior. This must be communicated, however, within the context of an empathic appreciation of the patient's urgent needs and difficulties in managing his or her feelings and impulses, which can reach suicidal proportions. Likewise, it may be important for even the self psychological therapist to represent reality at times, in order to help patients whose ego functioning is quite disturbed to expand their perceptions of a given situation. Empathic understanding may need to encompass the appreciation of how threatened or unworthy some patients feel in the face of interpersonal closeness or sensitivity. More thought needs to be given to the stage in treatment before a very disturbed borderline patient develops a stable, selfobject transference. While this period may be quite lengthy for some individuals, a self psychological approach still can be used. The therapist must move between knowing when "to wait it out" and when to interpret the patient's fears or resistance about entering a more intense therapeutic relationship. Paradoxically, being empathic in some instances—with more schizoid patients, for example—may mean that one should show restraint. Helping some patients to feel safe may be the most empathic stance. With others, however, empathic understanding may need to be augmented by actual selfobject responsiveness. The therapist must fulfill rather than merely understand selfobject needs.

The self psychological therapist's attempts to understand how his or her failures in empathic attunement have been experienced by the patient and to interpret how disruptions in the treatment relationship link up with traumatic aspects of the patient's childhood experiences have a powerful effect that enables patients to feel validated and cared for rather than blamed for their unrealistic and immature needs and reactions. A potential pitfall of these interventions with some patients, however, is that the therapist's assumption of responsibility for empathic failures may serve to ignore highly provocative and sadistic behavior or generate guilt over angry feelings in the presence of someone who is so "good." While narcissistic rage reactions are frequent when there are disruptions of the selfobject transference, it may be difficult for some patients to stay with their angry feelings without turning them against themselves. What may seem like a repair of the disruption may mask a depressive solution. The therapeutic interaction thus may replay the early child–parent relationship in which the child did not feel entitled to being or staying angry with a self-sacrificing parent.

Because of its radically different view of personality and pathology, self psychological treatment does not directly attempt to support the ego or to modify entrenched pathological defenses and internalized object relations. The belief that the ego and self can be strengthened sufficiently without the therapist's active support on the one hand, and his or her attempts to modify entrenched negative introjects on the other, is questionable. Self psychological treatment can embody interventions that address the clinical manifestations of this pathology within an empathic framework, but this model has not been elaborated on fully.

In its view of aggression and narcissistic rage as reactive rather than as a primary expression of drive, self psychology has often been criticized for using interventions that suppress or ignore a patient's pathological anger. The self psychologists refute this notion and respond that certain types of confrontations and interpretations provoke aggressive reactions. To argue this point is to enter into the long-standing and unresolved debate as to which view of human nature is more accurate. What seems more pertinent clinically is that there are borderline patients whose rage, whether it be primary or reactive, is so pervasive and sadistic toward others and the self that it does not easily yield to empathic interventions. Therapists begin to feel helpless and sometimes abused or controlled. Negative therapeutic reactions are common. Sometimes these patients show chronic suicidal or other types of extreme and dangerous behavior. Therapists of all persuasions are taxed by their unrelenting pathology. They require steadfastness and dedication on the part of the therapist and often hospitalization at certain points in the treatment.

Adler and Buie's Model

In putting forth a model that combines features of numerous approaches, Adler and Buie have attempted to overcome some of the problems associated with a rigid and single-minded treatment model. Their approach reflects an appreciation of the need for: a stable but flexible holding environment to help borderline individuals contain their overwhelming subjective experience of aloneness, panic, and rage in the face of separation or fears of abandonment; limits on potentially destructive behavior; empathic interpretations that help them overcome their fears of developing a selfobject transference; the fulfilling of selfobject functions and experiences of optimal disillusionment that lead to reparative experiences and the development of new, more positive internalizations and necessary psychic structures; and selective confrontations and interpretations of maladaptive defenses, self-defeating patterns, or destructive behavior. This model is the most responsive to borderline patients' needs for supports that will help them feel sustained during the difficult process of treatment, and the most demanding of therapists with respect to their flexibility and availability.

Adler and Buie's approach has a broad application across the borderline spectrum. They see the lack of evocative memory, which is caused by insufficient maternal holding experiences, not only in lower level borderline individuals but also underlying many defensive operations seen in the allegedly higher functioning borderline patients. Because they understand the problems that make it difficult for patients to form selfobject transferences, their approach focuses specifically on how to engage and sustain them. It can be used successfully with highly impulsive patients because of the combined use of empathy, holding, limits, structure, and confrontation when necessary. The use of interpretive as well as reparative techniques enables both an understanding of maladaptive patterns and new relationship experiences.

While this approach is very appealing because of its efforts at integration, it poses several problems. It is more difficult to use in practice than it seems in principle. The need to shift back and forth between basically different types of techniques in the treatment requires enormous flexibility and versatility on the part of the therapist. Empathy and confrontation cannot be used together easily without jeopardizing the selfobject transference. The fulfilling of various selfobject functions does not immediately result in a smooth treatment process. The intensity of the regression that ensues can ultimately have enormous potential therapeutic benefit, but it also stimulates frustrated wishes and yearnings that can be quite frightening to the patient, if not to the therapist. Empathic failures and disruptions are often very tumultuous and separations can necessitate periods of hospitalization. In the absence of professional supports for this type of approach, the therapist must be firm in his or her ability to withstand "the heat" engendered by non-traditional interventions.

RECONCILING THE CONFLICT AND
DEFICIT MODELS

There have been two main approaches to reconciling the conflict and deficit developmental and treatment models. Stolorow and Lachmann (1980) and the Blancks (1974, 1979) advocate a two-tier view of development, in which issues of deficit or a lower level of structuralization of the ego are on the lower end of a continuum, and problems of structural conflict or a more advanced level of structuralization of the ego are on the higher end. Treatment varies as a consequence of where a particular patient fits on this continuum. In contrast to this view, Eagle (1984) takes the position that the conflict and deficit models are merely two different ways of interpreting data and involve a false dichotomy. Conflict and deficit are always present and influence one another. Consequently, he opposes thinking of treatment in a dual way, although he seems biased in favor of a more traditional conflict-based treatment model.

While the two-tier approach has the appeal of giving equal weight to the important differences embodied in the conflict and deficit models, it oversimplifies the growth process. Individuals do not evolve from less structure to more structure *in toto*. There are different developmental lines that have their own unique timetables and eventually intersect. At the same time, adaptively functioning people are unique and do not necessarily show the same developmental achievements. Eagle's view of the conflict and deficit controversy as a false dichotomy makes an important point in drawing attention to the sometimes interlocking nature of developmental issues. He basically is opposed to a deficit model of development and treatment, however, and thus minimizes the unique contributions that the deficit perspective makes to understanding and treating severe disturbances.

Another approach to attempting to reconcile the conflict and deficit model involves the utilization of an integrative perspective such as the one suggested by Pine (1988) in his discussion of the place of the psychologies of drive, ego, object relations, and self in clinical understanding and treatment. In suggesting that each of these major points of view has its place in development, and that they should be used flexibly as tools in treatment, Pine moves beyond being wedded to one theoretical framework and treatment model.

An integrative perspective in the treatment of borderline disorders that utilizes different approaches in an individualized way rests on the view that no one theoretical formulation does justice to the complexity of personality development. Various explanatory frameworks are necessary to fully understand the diversity of borderline conditions and their treatment. It is the fit between a particular approach and a given patient's developmental needs that should guide the nature of the intervention. A range of techniques may be used.

GUIDING PRINCIPLES OF AN
INTEGRATIVE PERSPECTIVE

A Flexible Treatment Framework

The argument that borderline patients require a clear and firm treatment structure to help them to deal with their inner chaos has been made repeatedly by Kernberg and others. It is noteworthy, however, that Waldinger and Gunderson's (1987) presentation of successful psychotherapies of borderline individuals, each conducted by a therapist of a different persuasion, recounts many episodes in which patients managed to disregard the established structure even when the therapists were reasonably firm in their approach. One particular patient, who called frequently outside of appointment times despite the therapist's attempts to limit this behavior, was able to obtain an invitation for dinner at the therapist's home during a storm, and arrived unannounced at his vacation home where a session was granted. One could say that the therapist was inconsistent or inadequate in his limit-setting, or one could entertain the idea the patient persisted in getting what she needed from the therapist, who ultimately became responsive to her despite his own theoretical bias.

In stressing the importance of the therapist's availability to borderline patients between sessions, and even during vacations and other times of separation, Adler and Buie take a different position than does Kernberg. They depart from the traditional reliance on a fixed, unwavering schedule of appointments for designated amounts of time with no additional contact of any kind permitted. Likewise, in their attempts to create a more human and empathic ambience in the treatment, the self psychological group also move away from some of the stricter mores that have governed therapeutic decorum.

While the therapist's stability and consistency always are important in helping patients who lack self- and object-constancy, the treatment framework should be flexible and geared to each particular patient's needs. This may mean that a firm, or perhaps even rigid structure is indicated on the one hand, or that easy access to the therapist between sessions is permitted, if not encouraged, on the other. It is easy to lose sight of the fact that the details of the treatment framework that we therapists establish are generally based on dogma as well as on our own usually legitimate professional and personal needs rather than on the needs of patients. That we arrange, for instance: 45-minute sessions; fixed appointment times week after week, month after month, sometimes year after year; month-long (August) and even longer vacations; conference and lecture trips; particular fees and timely payments; and non-interference of our leisure or otherwise occupied time, may or may not be beneficial to our patients. This is the way we manage our lives and careers. We expect patients to cope with the structure we create. At times these reality demands will impose hardships on our patients, who are not wrong or too demanding for wanting or needing more from us. It may not be possible to provide daily contact with some patients or a telephone number when we are on vacation, but that patients might request such arrangements is understandable. Some may even require such contact in order to manage their feelings and impulses. At the very least, the therapist should be able to entertain the idea that borderline patients' frequent requests for something different or extra may reflect what they need rather than represent infantile demands or resistance.

Certain borderline patients can benefit from the establishment of strict guidelines and/or routines to help them maintain control of potentially destructive behavior and to take greater responsibility for their actions. This type of "contracting" should be a mutual process, with room for experimentation about what is effective rather than an unilateral and fixed statement about the patient's activities or about what the patient must or must not do.

The Importance of Empathy

Empathy is not the sole domain of the self psychologist, but Kohut and his followers have made an important contribution to the theory of treatment in their replacement of the therapists's functioning as an objective and expert observer with the therapist's immersion in the patient's subjective experience. Not only does this alter the ambience of the therapeutic relationship, it also radically alters the process by which the therapist understands the patient's feelings and behavior and attempts to intervene. Borderline patients, however, do not make it easy for the therapist to empathize with them because their inner experience is often chaotic and rapidly fluctuating. Consequently, Kernberg stresses that empathy should encompass patients' split off aggression and contradictory or disavowed self- and object-representations, as well as what they present at the manifest level at any given time. His technique, however, involves confrontation, which rarely is experienced empathically by the patient. It is important that those who work with borderline patients recognize and address their contradictory and changing internal states, but it is generally preferable to do so in an exploratory way that stays close to what the patient is able to acknowledge, rather than to confront and interpret the patient's reactions as evidence of defenses.

Establishment of a Holding Environment

The question of how best to help borderline individuals to contain their characteristic anxiety, impulsiveness, and self-destructiveness is an important one. Kernberg's use of limits, external structuring of the patient's life when necessary, and confrontation of primitive defenses and self-defeating or potentially harmful behavior, constitutes one type of holding environment. The Blancks's use of real object experiences and ego building techniques and Brandchaft and Stolorow's employment of empathic understanding reflect other ways of enabling patients to maintain control, a sense of connection, and self-cohesion. Adler and Buie's combined emphasis on therapist availability, empathic understanding and responsiveness, the use of transitional objects, selected confrontation, and limits and external structure when necessary, reflects their view of the complexity of the problem facing both patient and therapist. Other clinicians have suggested that selectively revealing personal information, such as particular interests or a vacation address, can serve an important "holding" function, and have recommended that the patient write down thoughts and feelings during periods of separation or use fantasy and visualization experiences involving the therapist in order to soothe themselves (Wells & Glickauf-Hughes, 1986).

Unfortunately, borderline patients' lack of object constancy or evocative memory and their intense rage, which makes them feel alone and alienated, often make it difficult for them to be "held" sufficiently by a therapist's empathy, accessibility, or realness. This is particularly true early in the treatment when a positive therapeutic relationship has not yet firmly developed or later during times of disruption. The patient's actual life circumstances also may present stresses that stimulate their impulsiveness and that overshadow the therapeutic holding environment, especially at the beginning of treatment. These factors create the need for more active and protective interventions, such as the use of limits and external structure. Likewise, some patients will utilize defenses to deal with their anger that weaken their sense of connection to others, including the therapist. Pointing out and reinforcing their positive feelings and ties is preferable to confronting their defenses generally, although this latter technique may be necessarily in selective instances.

To the degree that limits and structure are needed, it is important for the therapist to maintain empathy with patients and to engage them collaboratively in a problem-solving effort about what will enable them to contain their impulses and self-destructive behavior. Obviously, crises may occur that call for decisive action, but all too often therapists set limits unilaterally and arbitrarily in anger or frustration. Likewise, while some patients will tend to experience even the most gentle confrontation of their defenses or their potentially dangerous or self-defeating patterns as an attack, the therapist can take responsibility for communicating concern in non-assaultive and respectful ways. There is a subtle but important difference between telling a patient of one's worries about the extent of his or her drinking and informing the patient that he or she is showing denial in the face of alcohol abuse.

Differential Approach to Transference

While Kernberg and Masterson focus on the manifestations of the borderline individual's object-relations pathology and primitive defenses as they emerge in the transference, the Blancks, the self psychological group, and Adler and Buie stress the borderline's search for real objects, selfobjects, and positive holding objects in the therapeutic relationship. Rather than confront and interpret idealization or sudden shifts from idealization to devaluation, for example, as signs of splitting, they would allow such idealization to develop and would attempt to empathically repair disruptions and resultant narcissistic rage that might occur. Kernberg argues that this latter approach results in the therapist's denial of and/or collusion with the patient's aggression. Brandchaft and Stolorow retort that Kernberg's confrontations and interpretations produce aggressive patient responses. This polarized view does not capture the multifaceted nature of borderline patients' transferences that require differential interventions. Likewise, it is not sufficient to see the varying relationship paradigms that occur as a simple function of whether the patient is a lower or higher level borderline. The same individual may reflect different developmental issues at varying points in the treatment. This requires that the therapist perform the difficult task of understanding the patient's transferences flexibly and responding sensitively to what seems dominant at a particular time.

A Role for Support and Gratification

Support and gratification are different, although they may accompany one another. Support involves deliberate efforts to build up certain personality functions and structures. Gratification implies the meeting of patient needs. While Kernberg takes an extreme point of view about the importance of the therapist's maintenance of technical neutrality and abstinence to the exclusion of support and gratification, most of the other theorists who have been discussed are also quite cautious about this issue. Masterson and Rinsley advocate support only for the patient's appropriate efforts at individuation. The Blancks, while utilizing ego supportive measures extensively, believe that it is only when patients are "sick enough" that some of their needs may be gratified. In their emphasis on empathic understanding rather than optimal responsiveness, most but not all self psychologists stop short of fulfilling selfobject functions. Only Adler and Buie's approach takes a clearly positive position on the importance of the therapist in gratifying selfobject needs.

It is beyond the scope of this chapter to review all of the reasons that the American psychoanalytic community has relegated supportive measures to a second class position vis à vis insight-oriented techniques, and viewed abstinence and technical neutrality as superior to gratification and support. If a treatment includes supportive techniques, it is considered to be psychotherapy rather than psychoanalysis. These issues have more to do with values and psychoanalytic dogma, however, than with what has been shown to be important in child development or efficacious in helping patients.

Mounting evidence from studies of children shows that new behavior is acquired in various ways. This challenges the view that frustration is essential to growth. Likewise, there is no scientific basis for the belief that meeting patients' needs suppresses their anger or makes them too dependent, regressed, fixated, incapable of internalization, unable to develop transferences, or unwilling to focus on self-understanding. It is highly moralistic to argue that it is permissible to gratify patients only when they are at the more disturbed end of the health/illness spectrum. This implies that healthier individuals are not entitled to having their needs met, that gratification will harm them in some way, and that maturity means having to tolerate more frustration. The creation in therapy of an adult version of those factors and processes that foster normal development early in life can bring new power to the therapeutic relationship for all patients.

It is true that a therapist who maintains a position of technical neutrality and abstinence has a clearer road map with respect to the nature of his or her interventions than does the therapist who attempts to support or gratify the patient. The very uncharted nature of this territory makes for uncertainty and error. Patients who have suffered early deprivations do not experience being given to easily. Turbulence and disruptions are frequent as early childhood yearnings are revived.

We lack criteria for when one does what to whom? Most of what has been written on this subject points out or illustrates the pitfalls of a therapist's well-intentioned but inappropriate use of support, gratification, and reparenting (Chatham, 1985, pp. 389-390; Druck, 1989, pp. 355-360). The assumption is often made that meeting patients' needs is a form of countertransference acting-out. It is difficult to refute this view if support and gratification are always regarded negatively in expressive psychotherapy or psychoanalysis. While there is a risk that therapists may be meeting their own needs to the detriment of their patients', this possibility exists in the use of any technique. There are dangers inherent in frustrating and confronting patients and reexposing them to deprivation and rejection.

Establishing a proper role for the use of support and gratification in psychotherapy, alongside other techniques generally and in the treatment of borderline individuals specifically, is what is important. The fact that so much attention has been focused on the possible harm resulting from giving too much rather than from giving too little reflects the deep-seated prohibition against gratification that is embedded in religious and societal as well as professional values. This has led to a skewed framing of the issue. Instead of asking when it is not beneficial to meet patients' needs, the question has been turned around. When the psychoanalytic establishment moves beyond its preoccupation with the detrimental effects of giving to patients, it will be possible to develop a better understanding of when and when not to meet patient needs, and of what types of gratification and support are beneficial or harmful.

A Role for Reparative Experiences

The argument that therapy can never substitute for poor parenting has been used by many clinicians to minimize the importance of positive experiences in the treatment relationship that can serve as a basis for identification, internalization, amelioration of deficits, and structural change. An emphasis on the content of therapeutic interventions takes precedence over relational experiences that may be emotionally corrective and reparative. Helping patients to understand the origins and nature of their pathology is given priority over trying to develop a treatment environment that nurtures development. The dangers, rather than the benefits, of reparenting are emphasized. Kernberg's treatment epitomizes this view, while all of the other approaches that have been described depart from it more or less. Masterson and Rinsley, the Blancks, Kohut and the other self psychologists, and Buie and Adler all show some appreciation of the therapeutic power of the treatment experience or process in addition to, and in some instances, instead of, its content per se, but are careful to say that they are not advocating reparenting.

In the treatment of the diverse group of borderline disorders the issue should not be whether or not to use the therapeutic relationship reparatively but how best to do so. To the degree that borderline individuals do not share exactly the same constitutional endowments, caretaking experiences, environmental supports, and developmental deficits, they require an individualized treatment approach that is fitted to their specific needs. This places special demands on the therapist in the treatment itself, and in the professional community, where following a particular model is a matter of status and acceptance.

Modification of Negative Introjects and Pathological Defenses

Arguing that it is not *actual* objects that are taken in, Kernberg attributes problems in internalized object relations to the individual's drives that influence the ways in which external experiences are perceived and assimilated. Masterson and Rinsley address a limited aspect of internalized object-relations pathology in their description of the rewarding and withdrawing split object-relations part-unit that stems from the mother's actual responses to the child's efforts at separation–individuation. The Blancks's ego building approach is aimed at those patients who have not consolidated internal structure and attempts to develop new structures. Kohut and other self psychologists focus on the self rather than object relations but the connection between these two lines of development is not clearly conceptualized. Adler and Buie address the absence of positive holding introjects rather than the presence of negative ones.

There are borderline individuals who show internalized object-relations pathology that is often accompanied by intense and unrelenting self-destructive or self-defeating behavior, or an inability to free themselves from the negative and sometimes unconscious internal voices or scripts of the past that control their current behavior. These internalizations are based largely on *real* experiences with others, although the process of internalization is complex and clearly does bear some relationship to what the child brings to his or her transactions with the world. The therapist must help patients to become aware of the deleterious introjects that dominate their behavior, and which are generally syntonic — that is, the individual experiences them as a part of his or her personality. Pathological defenses such as splitting protect these introjects. When the therapist tries to focus on their presence to help free patients from their power, patients often respond as if the therapist is attacking them and resist. Indeed, this is true to the extent that the therapist is opposing not only a defense by external objects that have become internalized as parts of the self. Even when these negative internalizations become more alien, they still exert enormous pressure. An approach that does not blame the patient for the presence of this pathology is needed. This can be accomplished by empathically relating to the conditions of early life that led to the patient's identification with and internalization of selected parts of those individuals who opposed the development of his or her unique self. The therapist also shows the patient how his or her attitudes and behavior continue to reflect these early influences. A focus on the presence and influence of negative introjects may lead to disruptions in the therapeutic relationship that will need to be repaired. This emphasis also must be accompanied by efforts to strengthen the self by enabling new, more positive internalizations to develop. In an application of Fairbairn's work to the treatment of borderline disorders, Seinfeld (1990) has recently put forth a promising new synthesis of techniques to help patients to relinquish their "bad" objects.

Expansion of the Content of Interpretation

All of the approaches that have been discussed utilize explanatory or interpretive techniques. They differ, however, in the content, form, and style of what is interpreted. For example, Kernberg's authoritative interpretaions focus on the role of aggression in the borderline individual's pathology. Masterson and Rinsley address fears of abandonment and regressive longings, while the Blancks's interpretations are directed at the patient's highest level of ego functioning and are offered more tentatively. The self psychological group and Adler and Buie focus on the deficiencies in empathy in the patient's early caretaking environment and their impact.

Not all borderline patients reflect only one core issue, and the same patient may show more than one key dynamic at different times in the treatment. A therapist who is wedded to one way of hearing and understanding the material runs the risk of serious misattunement. This does not mean that the therapist should refrain from ordering what the patient is saying or should start each session *de novo*. The therapist, however, must remain open-minded. As Pine (1988, pp. 576–577) indicates in his discussion of Freud's famous guideline that the therapist should listen with "evenly hovering attention" to the patient's associations, "the intent of evenly hovering attention is not to produce blank minds, but uncommitted ones—minds receptive to the organization of this particular content in this particular hour in ways true to its potentially unique offering."

Therapist Responsibility for Countertransference

While the treatment approaches that have been described in this book emphasize different aspects of countertransference, there is a general consensus that therapists are especially vulnerable to problematic reactions that can obstruct the treatment when working with borderline individuals because of the impact of the patient's pathology. The degree to which therapists should use their own reactions as diagnostic clues to what patients are experiencing is a debatable issue. While projective defenses may be powerful in many instances and may need to be understood and addressed, to say that a patient is "inducing" a particular response in the therapist blames a patient for an unconscious mechanism and is risky. It shifts the responsibility for the therapist's reactions to the patient. While an individual's provocative and even obnoxious behavior may result in a therapist's feeling angry, helpless, or wanting to withdraw, the patient has not caused the therapist to react in these ways. Countertransference is the responsibility of the therapist. A therapist's own responses may be a clue that the patient is struggling with similar feelings that are being projected. They may also, however, indicate either that the therapist's own unresolved issues are at work and/or that the therapist has unwittingly stimulated a patient's negative reactions by an insensitive remark or other type of empathic failure. To readily conclude that the patient is making the therapist experience certain feelings because of his or her internal pathology is too one-sided a view of the nature of the patient–therapist interaction. It assumes that the therapist has no effect on the patient's reactions. At the same time, patients do bring their experiences in past human relationships with them, and their characteristic responses may have some degree of autonomy from external triggers. Their urgent needs and pathological defenses do exert enormous force in the therapeutic interaction. This is a complex issue and all of its facets need to be carefully considered in the clinical situation.

Assessment and Treatment of the Family and Social Environment

In their emphasis on individual treatment, all of the models that have been described have not sufficiently conceptualized the ongoing role of interpersonal and environmental factors in either aggravating and perpetuating borderline disorders or in the treatment process. While the borderline individual's internalized pathology results in structures and deficits that shape the way the external world is experienced, close interpersonal relationships and the supports or constraints presented by the social environment may nurture or obstruct positive change. Consequently, diagnosis must consider the borderline individual's environmental context, and in many instances treatment should include work with the couple, the family, and other members of the patient's social network (Goldstein, 1983). The exact nature of this combined treatment approach will be discussed in later chapters.

CONCLUSION

This chapter has discussed some of the strengths and limitations of five major treatment approaches and has concluded that there is not an optimal model for all borderline individuals. My consideration of the issue of whether the conflict and deficit models can be reconciled has suggested an integrative perspective in which the diverse approaches can be drawn upon as they seem to best fit the patient's developmental needs. The principles guiding such a perspective involve: (1) a flexible treatment framework; (2) the importance of empathy; (3) the establishment of a holding environment; (4) a differential approach to transference; (5) a role for support and gratification; (6) a role for reparative experiences; (7) modification of negative introjects and pathological defenses; (8) expansion of the content of interpretation; (9) therapist responsibility for countertransference; and (10) assessment and treatment of the family and social environment.

9

Hospital Treatment

While the majority of borderline individuals are treated in the community, a sizable number are admitted to hospitals at least once and sometimes repeatedly. Hospital stays are usually short-term and follow suicide attempts, psychotic episodes, escalating alcohol and/or drug abuse, life-threatening eating disorders, or other types of destructive behavior. Treatment focuses on resolving the immediate crises that lead to the hospitalization. Some borderline patients, however, undergo longer and more intensive hospital treatment. While sharing some common features and problems, the short- and long-term hospital treatment models are quite different. Because it is difficult to integrate both approaches in one structure, often hospital units and in some instances, entire facilities, provide one or the other form of treatment. This chapter will consider the overlapping and differential characteristics of both the short- and long-term hospital treatment models.

THE NEED FOR HOSPITALIZATION

In instances in which a borderline patient's escalating behavior requires hospital admission, some clinicians favor a highly focused short-term approach on both clinical and practical grounds. They argue that long-term hospitalization increases problematic behavior, overgratifies dependency needs, stimulates regressive yearnings, and weakens ego functioning (Friedman, 1975; Nurnberg & Suh, 1978). As hospitalizations are increasingly short-term, it is important to design briefer treatments that return patients to the community more able to function than previously.

Short-term hospitalization of approximately 1 month: (1) offers thorough diagnostic evaluations; (2) helps patients, families, and sometimes out-patient therapists, over crisis periods; (3) begins treatment; and (4) connects patients to community resources and to longer-term out-patient treatment that may have more ambitious goals. In these instances, after-care is necessary in order to prevent further hospitalization and chronicity and to promote more adaptive functioning.

While the problems or events that lead to the borderline individual's need for hospitalization generally are acute, they arise in the context of entrenched personality pathology which is difficult to alter quickly. Because borderline individuals tend to be chronically unstable, suicidal, self-destructive, or antisocial, brief hospitalizations often fall short of modifying their basic difficulties. They remain vulnerable to repeated crises and marginal functioning. Those who cannot sustain themselves even minimally in the community without endangering themselves or others may be transferred to "protective" or custodial public settings, but often are quickly discharged and do not receive appropriate follow-up care. Some clincians favor a long-term intensive hospital treatment approach that aims at modifying the borderline individual's core pathology.

Long-term hospitalizations of 6–18 months are indicated on clinical grounds for those borderline patients who are so chronically self-destructive or disorganized in their functioning that they cannot be maintained outside of a structured setting, and/or who need support and protection during the periods of intense regression that are stimulated by intensive psychotherapy. The first type of patient usually shows pervasive problems in, or repeated, severe sudden losses of impulse control, chronic suicidal or self-mutilating behavior, habitual substance abuse, negative therapeutic reactions, low motivation for treatment, antisocial features, and chaotic or highly pathological family and social environments that offer few supports for more adaptive behavior. While brief hospitalizations may be used at extremely dangerous points with such individuals, the crisis-ridden nature of their lives keeps them perpetually at risk. Day hospitals or out-patient programs that offer frequent contact and structure might be sufficient for some of the less acting-out of these patients, but unfortunately such services are sorely lacking. Those that do exist tend to focus on the schizophrenic population, who have different treatment needs. The second type of patient, who generally functions at a higher level than those in the former group, experiences intense panic and emptiness at times, usually because of transference disruptions or significant losses or disappointments in their lives that activate suicidal and other forms of self-destructive behavior. Brief hospitalizations often can sustain them during these crises, but long-term hospital treatment may provide the necessary structure that some of these patients need to enable them to tolerate the intensity and turbulence of intensive psychotherapy.

From a practical point of view, only a small segment of those borderline individuals who might benefit from long-term hospitalization actually receive it because of financial considerations. Even when patients and their families possess the financial assets or insurance to pay for such a costly treatment, it is undertaken as a last resort when out-patient efforts have repeatedly failed or are continually disrupted by emergencies or frequent short-term hospitalizations.

THE NATURE OF THE THERAPEUTIC MILIEU

Intensive long-term hospital treatment provides more than a protective or custodial structure. While there are different philosophies of hospital treatment, they share the view that the in-patient setting should be designed so that it provides a therapeutic milieu for the borderline patient. Along with psychotherapy and other treatment modalities and adjunct therapies, such an environment aims at the modification or amelioration of selected aspects of the borderline individual's core pathology. Kernberg and Adler, two main proponents of the hospital treatment of borderline patients, emphasize different features of the therapeutic milieu that are consistent with their general treatment approaches as described in Chapters 6 and 7.

Diagnosing Internalized Object-Relations Pathology

Kernberg (1976, 1984) sees long-term hospitalization as helping borderline patients with needed controls while simultaneously enabling staff to diagnose and treat their internalized object-relations pathology. As patients interact with others, their split self- and object-representations will become apparent. For example, a male patient might idealize his primary therapist to whom he relates in an admiring and pleasant manner, while at the same time he devalues the head nurse whom he treats with contempt and anger. Interpersonal relationships on the unit will reflect a variety of such themes. Kernberg sees these developments as stemming largely from the projection of "good" and "bad" self- and object-representations into the environment, rather than as understandable reactions to the "real" qualities of the those in the outside world. There may be kernels of reality to some of the patient's perceptions, however, since they tend to seek out and relate to certain staff members because of their particular characteristics. Borderline individuals also have the uncanny ability to sense and exacerbate latent staff conflict, and they selectively distort and exaggerate others' characteristics for their own purposes unconsciously (Gabbard, 1989). By identifying their own reactions and understanding what is being projected, the staff can gather a picture of the inner world of the patient that can be used by the patient's primary therapist to confront and interpret his or her internalized object-relations pathology. In fact, a patient's interactions in the therapeutic milieu themselves can be used to diagnose the presence of a borderline disorder when the diagnosis seems unclear (Bauer et al., 1980).

In Kernberg's view, nurses, attendants, and other therapeutic personnel must provide an environment that is clear and consistent in its expectations, discipline, and granting of privileges. The clarity and stability of this structure both helps patients and provides a baseline against which their internalized pathology can be diagnosed. At the same time, the structure should be sufficiently flexible to permit appropriate outlets for and learning experiences in the regulating of impulses and other ego functions, and to enable patients to "show their true colors." The hospital unit should not be an authoritarian structure. Rather, it should provide patients with meaningful participation in decisions and activities that pertain to the quality of life in the hospital and that foster improved ego functioning. Community meetings, patient government, task-oriented groups, as well as school, occupational, and other types of adjunct therapies are part of an optimal therapeutic community.

An important requirement of this type of setting is that staff must refrain from colluding with the patient's projections and from acting-out their countertransference reactions. Staff must be educated in how to recognize and deal with splitting. They must be aware of how patients relate to them and recognize what feelings are being stirred up. When patient–staff interactions are experienced as too "real," staff conflict and countertransference acting-out occur. The most common manifestation of this problem is when staff become polarized. Seemingly "good" staff members fight with those who are "bad" about the accuracy of their perceptions of and management of the patient. Therapeutic stalemates and premature discharges can occur. Staff–patient meetings, rounds, and team meetings can provide opportunities for all those involved in the care of patients to share their impressions and to plan individualized treatment strategies. An atmosphere of openness and reflection is important.

There are several problems inherent in Kernberg's conception of the therapeutic milieu. Since it focuses on how the patient recreates his or her internal pathology in the environment and on what the patient is doing to "induce" staff to respond in certain ways, this view minimizes the role of staff attitudes and behavior in provoking patients. It assumes that basic human concern, limits, and firmness are sufficient in treating borderline patients and does not consider the degree to which many of these individuals may require a more nurturing and ego-building milieu. The approach is clear but rigid, and does not allow for sufficient individualization. In attempting to address the patient's use of splitting, projective identification, and other primitive defenses, it risks creating another type of split in which the patients are "bad" and the staff are "good."

Providing a Holding Environment

Adler (1985) emphasizes the hospital milieu's "good enough" mothering and holding functions for borderline individuals who are desperate, panicky, and who experience overwhelming aloneness and intense rage. The therapeutic environment should be empathic and soothing as well as structured and controlled. It must help patients to feel understood, safe, and secure while they attempt to understand what leads to their intense distress that often threatens their survival, and to acquire newer, more positive internalizations and capacities.

While Adler's conception of the therapeutic milieu contains more nurturing elements than does Kernberg's, this does not mean that staff should always be warm and giving since these responses may stimulate or perpetuate more regressive behavior. Limits and firmness may be necessary, but their use should be individualized according to the developmental needs of the patients and not used punitively in the face of a patient's provocative behavior. Too great an emphasis on the control of behavior and the confrontation of defenses will escalate rather than diffuse aggressive outbursts or self-destructive behavior. Empathy for the turbulent and frightening nature of the patient's inner experience of aloneness and abandonment also helps to contain the patient's impulses through its soothing effects.

In keeping with his emphasis on the building up of new, more positive internalizations, Adler points to the need for staff to lend themselves for this purpose. He also stresses the importance of providing a full range of opportunities for patients to strengthen their sense of autonomy and appropriate ego functioning. Pointing out the problems of collaboration and countertransference acting-out in the hospital treatment of borderline patients, Adler recognizes the importance of helping staff to understand and internalize the treatment philosophy, and to have ample opportunity for and support in discussing and managing their usually intense reactions to patients. Structures that foster open communication are necessary so that staff can understand the ways in which certain patients may be stimulating countertransference feelings.

The main difficulty with Adler's approach is not in its conception but in its implementation. It requires that staff be highly individualizing and flexible in treatment planning and interventions, and allows for more diversity within the milieu. This can stimulate uncertainty and divisiveness among hospital personnel about how best to treat a particular patient, especially when the patient's behavior escalates despite staff efforts to be empathic and responsive. The staff need a good deal of support and conviction to carry out their work. This approach, however, has the potential to overcome the we–they atmosphere between patients and staff, and to be more attuned to the special and varying needs of the borderline population.

THE TREATMENT STRUCTURE

A common practice, particularly in teaching hospitals, involves the use of teams composed of those staff who work directly with and who are responsible for the overall planning and management of the treatment of a particular patient. Each member on the team, which is often interdisciplinary, has a unique role in the patient's care. This model requires a high degree of collaboration and mutual respect. Each patient usually has a medical or non-medical primary therapist, a social worker who works with the family and is involved in the patient's transition to the community, a nurse who oversees the patient's life on the unit, and an activities or occupational therapist. One person coordinates the team's efforts and may have final decision-making authority.

Other models do exist, for example, one in which the primary therapist has responsibility for work with the patient, the family, and other aspects of the case. This has the advantage of reducing the need for collaboration, which can be time-consuming and fraught with interpersonal tension. It may not be advantageous in certain instances, such as when the separation of therapeutic functions may be optimal or necessary, nor does it allow for as much specialized expertise as does the interdisciplinary team model.

In many settings the primary therapist has responsibility not only for the psychotherapy but also for decisions about the patient's privileges, status on the unit, passes, disciplinary measures, and so on. This model helps to convey the message that the patient's life on the unit is not separate from but a crucial part of the therapy. The success of this approach, however, rests on the therapist's respect for the observations and opinions of other staff who interact with the patient and on his or her ability to seek out and integrate their views when working with a particular patient. A potential disadvantage for the therapist is the time-consuming nature of having to negotiate the passes and privileges of volatile and provocative patients.

To remedy the problems in collaboration and to free the primary therapist to conduct the psychotherapy unhampered by the need to manage the patient's life, some settings have found it preferable to separate the administrative and therapeutic functions of the treatment. Typically, the nursing staff have the responsibility for the patient's life on the unit, and the therapist oversees the psychotherapy. This model results in clearer staff authority over the management of the unit, but presents certain risks. The primary therapist and nursing staff may each go their own, separate ways rather than work collaboratively with a particular patient. The patient may then attempt to "split" the nursing staff from the therapist, and the therapist may ignore rather than deal with the patient's interactions on the unit.

Another important and related consideration in hospital treatment is the setting's policy regarding the use of private or non-unit-based practitioners in the in-patient phase of treatment. In teaching centers the primary therapist is usually in training on the unit or a member of the full-time staff. If a patient has been in psychotherapy on an out-patient basis, or if an in-patient therapist has rotated off the unit, the therapist is not allowed to continue treating the patient, even if the therapist is affiliated with the setting. Thus, both short- and long-term hospitalizations may interrupt a preexisting treatment. The advantage of this policy is that the patient has an in-patient therapist who is present on and fully integrated into the milieu and who can participate easily in collaboration. When administrative and therapeutic functions are separated and mechanisms for collaboration are well-established, however, it is possible to integrate a non-hospital or non-unit-based therapist into the treatment in order to maintain continuity.

THE RELATIONSHIP TO THE FAMILY

The findings of Goldstein's (1979) study of the families of 30 borderline and schizophrenic adolescents and young adults who were hospitalized for one year clearly showed that the outcome of treatment for those patients whose families were involved in the hospitalization was much better than the outcome for those patients whose families were minimally involved. The degree of involvement was defined by the nature and amount of contact the family had with the social worker assigned to the case. It varied from minimal or no contact to an intensive program of family, multifamily group, and individual treatment. A related finding was that the patients whose parents were the most accepting of the hospitalization and the most able to grasp the seriousness of the patient's problems did better than those patients whose families were opposed to the hospitalization and who denied the nature of the patient's difficulties.

Based on her study, Goldstein concluded that the following components are important to successful long-term hospital treatment: (1) a high degree of family involvement; (2) efforts to help families develop a therapeutic alliance with the hospital; and (3) attempts to lessen family members' use of denial. In a later paper, Goldstein (1981) questioned some of the practices in hospital settings that may make the necessary collaboration between hospital and family more difficult, and suggested a more flexible approach to work with families.

Family members generally bring a sense of shame and guilt, low self-esteem, frustration, fatigue, helplessness, and hopelessness to interactions with hospital staff. Sometimes judgmental and non-supportive attitudes are communicated to such families and hospital policies and practices are insensitive to their needs. Families lack information and feel excluded from decisions, blamed, or at the mercy of the hospital's arbitrary authority. Fearing abandonment and loss of control and easily humiliated, borderline families are quite sensitive to separations and blows to their self-esteem. Their anxiety mobilizes denial, splitting, and projection as well as other dysfunctional responses. These reactions, in turn, lead hospital staff to feel that such families are highly pathological, difficult, and demanding. Maintaining empathy with them is difficult. A circular negative process gets established that obstructs efforts to improve the family's alliance with the hospital.

The family, as well as the borderline patient, requires a therapeutic holding environment that helps them to contain their anxiety and to become collaborators in the treatment process. An approach that is sensitive to the family's needs and defenses and that respects their rights as consumers is important to lessening their more extreme reactions and to developing a therapeutic alliance. Avoiding power struggles, providing information and access to professionals, and involving them in decision-making early in treatment helps in the engagement process. While many families may require treatment for their "pathology," they may perceive their psychological survival as being threatened by such efforts unless and until they feel supported. Without such support, the family's resistance and acting-out usually increases and undermines the treatment of the patient.

In some instances in which families are potentially or actually violent or flagrantly destructive, a more limit-setting and confrontative approach may be necessary. It can backfire, however, and lead to the family removing the patient from the hospital against medical advice. Its success will depend on the ability and authority of the therapist to implement limits and make them stick. It is also contingent on the degree of administrative support that the unit has from other important senior staff in the hospital to whom family members may complain. Limits and the use of confrontations may succeed in controlling the family's behavior long enough for the patient's individual treatment to take effect, but they do not promote a therapeutic alliance nor do they motivate the family to alter its dysfunctional patterns with which the patient has to continue to deal. It may alienate the family from professionals even further. This is problematic since most hospitalized patients continue to need their families for long periods of time both during and after hospitalization. Therapeutic personnel tend to overestimate the patient's ability to separate from even a highly pathological family emotionally and physically.

THE RELATIONSHIP TO THE COMMUNITY

In-patient settings rely on referrals from outside professionals and members of the community and must work to maintain positive relationships with these groups. When patients are admitted, it is possible to respectfully involve an outside therapist of the patient or family even if these individuals are not permitted to be part of the hospital treatment team. It should be expected that the patient and/or family will eventually return to this therapist, unless there are special and compelling reasons why this is contraindicated. Such therapists should always be contacted for information and invited to participate in conferences involving major treatment planning decisions. This is important on therapeutic grounds with borderline patients, who show such contradictory and changing behavior and who generally are not the most accurate historians. It is also common courtesy. Too often private therapists have the experience of being excluded or devalued by the hospital therapist and of having their patients "robbed" from them. Sometimes difficulties in implementing certain practical arrangements and changes in the patient's needs over time do obstruct collaboration or the patient's return to an outside therapist. There is an unfortunate tendency, however, for hospital-based staff to display a collective arrogance in which they view themselves as the "good" therapists and the outside world of professionals as the "bad" ones. They justify their negative reactions and behavior on the basis that the private therapist mishandled the case because of his or her countertransference or lack of specialized skills. This is especially true when the outside therapist is a non-medical professional and interdisciplinary rivalries are acted-out. Outside therapists themselves feel victimized or intimidated by the "bad" hospital and do not assert themselves. This is another way in which mental health professionals become vulnerable to the internal splitting and archaic selfobject needs of borderline patients.

Linkages to community organizations that permit expeditious admission and discharge planning need to be established. Education and consultation can play an important role in community relations, along with the hospital's participation in assessing the need for and planning of mental health services. Hospitals are too often viewed as ivory towers, isolated from and indifferent to the surrounding environment.

TREATMENT MODALITIES

Individual Psychotherapy

In hospitals or units that specialize in the long-term treatment of borderline patients, intensive individual psychotherapy is generally the main modality. While numerous psychotherapeutic models exist (as discussed in Chapters 6 and 7), often a setting will tend to utilize one dominant approach. The advantage of this is that both the psychotherapy and the milieu can be organized to embody and facilitate the goals and nature of a particular treatment model. Staff can be educated in this approach and can work together with a sense of clarity and common purpose. While this does not permit sufficient individualization when the dominant model is rather rigid and prescriptive, it is difficult for staff to create a milieu that embodies vastly different ways of treating patients. For example, a Kernbergian approach has very different requirements than a Kohutian or Adlerian model.

As different children in the same family need different kinds of parenting, it seems desirable for psychotherapy and milieu treatment to be sufficiently individualized and flexible to meet the diverse needs of the borderline population. When the use of different types of psychotherapy is permitted or encouraged, it is important that this be done thoughtfully rather than arbitrarily because a therapist or supervisor wants to experiment with or is wedded to a favorite model. Every attempt should be made to create a therapeutic milieu around a particular patient that is integrated with the goals and nature of that patient's psychotherapy. For example, if a therapist sees the patient's difficulties as stemming from a lack of soothing and positive introjects, it is important that the staff involved with the patient understand the patient's treatment needs, resolve differences of opinion about how to treat the patient, and gear their interventions accordingly. Otherwise, the psychotherapy and the hospital milieu may work at cross purposes with one another. The inevitable splitting that occurs becomes more intense around actual staff divisions, and the risk of staff polarization around a particular patient is likely. Sometimes this results in premature discharges as the staff cannot contain their own disagreements and tensions. The staff, who have to work together, unwittingly sacrifice the patient in order to restore some degree of harmony.

Integration and Nature of Family Treatment

There are different models for integrating family therapy into the overall treatment of hospitalized borderline patients. While Kernberg acknowledges that some work with the parents of borderline patients may be critical in order to keep family members from sabotaging individual treatment or from colluding with the patient's pathology, he does not favor the use of family treatment generally. Maintaining the traditional view that the transference between the patient and therapist should not be contaminated by the therapist's contact with others in the patient's life, he also explicitly warns against the primary therapist ever working with the family. Instead, he recommends using a separate therapist for the parents or family (Kernberg, 1979). Advocating the separation of patient and family in the beginning stages of hospitalization, Masterson (1972, 1976) advises against family treatment initially. While suggesting that mothers may need support early in the admission in order to help them tolerate their feelings of rage and abandonment, he reserves family sessions for later in the treatment. They may be used to help patients to separate from their families by recognizing the pathological transactions of which they are a part.

In contrast to both Kernberg and Masterson, Shapiro and his co-workers (1977) have proposed that family treatment be a vital part of the work with borderline adolescents and young adults from the beginning of hospitalization. They argue that conjoint family treatment generally fosters the formation of a therapeutic alliance with the identified patient. Ideally, couple sessions with the parents conducted by a separate therapist and conjoint family sessions in which the borderline patient's therapist and the parents' therapist come together should accompany individual treatment. Multiple family groups can be used also to help foster the therapeutic alliance with families, to help them contain their primitive defenses, and to facilitate mutual support and problem solving.

While Gunderson, Kerr, and Englund (1980) also believe that family therapy at the outset may be necessary with those families who are overinvolved and who cannot tolerate much separation, they recommend that family therapy should not be utilized initially with families who show neglect and underinvolvement. In these cases, family sessions heighten parental anxiety and blaming that may interfere with the development of a therapeutic alliance with the parents. They prefer to see the parents separately for a period for the purpose of support. Later, after an alliance has been established, family sessions may be useful to clarify family interactions.

A differential and flexible use of family treatment is indicated in clinical work with families of hospitalized borderline adolescents and young adults. Some form of parental involvement is important to the successful outcome of intensive hospital treatment (Goldstein, 1979), but the specific approach will vary with the particular family. In the initial stages of hospitalization, supportive treatment of the parents is necessary in order to foster a therapeutic alliance; to help them share their concerns about the patient's problems and hospitalization and to deal with the immediate crisis; to provide necessary information; to improve their self-esteem; to reduce their use of primitive defenses of splitting, denial, and projection that often lead to scapegoating of the patient and/or the hospital staff and to premature efforts to take the patient home; to enhance parental empathy; to facilitate problem solving; and to reduce internal and external stresses. It is useful for a particular staff member, usually a social worker, to be assigned to work with the parents and to be there for them. This paves the way for the use of a co-therapy model in which the patient's primary therapist and the parents' therapist or social worker meet together with the patient and the family when family sessions are scheduled. While the co-therapy model will necessitate that the patient's therapist manage his or her boundaries with the family and his relationship with the patient, more therapeutic mileage will be gained from this approach than will be lost. It enables the primary therapist to see family interactions directly and to better utilize these perceptions in the individual treatment of the patient. It also provides the patient with a ally who can validate his or her experiences in the family, helps to contain the family and gives support to the therapists, reduces collaborative tensions and the "splitting" of therapists by the patient and family, and promotes the integration of individual and family treatment. Exceptions to this practice are indicated when family members are extremely suspicious, overtly paranoid or psychotic, potentially violent and/or frankly cruel, or sociopathic. In some instances it may be possible to use one therapist for everyone, but this model often does not permit the safety, confidentiality, empathy, and individualization that many of the family members require.

The usual practice of discouraging families from communicating directly with the patient's therapist or with senior staff tends to escalate alliance problems. Whether out of caring or guilt, families generally feel that it is incumbent upon them to do the utmost to help their children. They also have problems in giving over their parenting functions to the hospital, and often feel an urgent need to speak to the primary therapist or a senior staff person in the beginning of treatment. Rather than viewing such a request as bypassing the staff member who has been assigned to work with the parents, staff should arrange a meeting of this kind. This will avoid an unnecessary power struggle at a fragile time in the treatment, diffuse anxiety and guilt, and help to establish a therapeutic alliance with the family. Similarly, a family's request to bring in a consultant should be granted and facilitated. Often an outside expert can relieve family anxiety and help them to support the hospital's treatment recommendations.

Generally, regular sessions with the parents alone are indicated in the early stages of treatment, but additional family sessions that include the patient and the primary therapist, if a co-therapy model is utilized, may be important with overinvolved families. Such meetings help to reduce separation anxiety and fears of abandonment. With more rejecting, idealizing, or denying families, however, family sessions usually are contraindicated initially as they tend to create defensiveness, withdrawal, and alliance problems. They should be reserved for later in the treatment when the parents are more open and less rigid. Orientation and lecture/discussion groups on topics of special interest to the parents, and multifamily meetings that provide support and promote problem solving also help to promote and sustain a therapeutic alliance with the family.

Early meetings with the family together help to provide a holding environment that contains the family's intense reactions, and enable the patient and the therapist to share an experience in which they can both observe the patient's role within the family and the nature of family interactions. All family members can get support. Attempts to clarify and modify dysfunctional family interactions can be made. It is important that family members feel safe to share their thoughts, feelings, and usual ways of behaving. The nature of the therapeutic task will vary. In some families confrontation and interpretation of splitting, projective identification, and other primitive defenses and destructive interactions and behaviors may be necessary. In other cases the focus may be on understanding the frustrated selfobject needs and ego and self deficits of family members and increasing empathic understanding and responsiveness. The nature of these differing approaches will be discussed in Chapter 10.

Group Therapy

Most clinicians have cautioned against the use of intensive group therapy for borderline individuals or have sometimes viewed it as a possible adjunct to rather than a substitute for individual psychotherapy. They argue that most borderline patients are not suited to this modality because of their excessive vulnerability, self-centeredness, impulsiveness, anxiety, and paranoia. Unstructured groups mobilize intense regression and stimulate volatility and primitive defenses in these patients. The use of groups is not limited, however, to intensive group therapy. Supportive, structured, and task-oriented groups can be used effectively with many borderline individuals. There are those who cannot tolerate the intensity of individual treatment and who do better in groups where their transference is diffused among the group members. In hospitals and out-patient settings supportive groups can be used to promote reality testing and other ego functions, self-esteem, and interpersonal relationships. They offer many opportunities for identification with and internalization of others. Task-oriented groups for discharge planning, the development of daily living or social skills, or for other special purposes can provide rich opportunities for borderline patients to learn to exercise their autonomy and to expand their ego and social functioning. Likewise, the nature of community living in a hospital setting is fertile ground for the formation of a patient government and ad hoc special interest groups (for example, to plan parties or to address problems that affect the patient community). These forums also enable patients to exercise their capacity for decision-making, problem-solving, and collaboration with others.

Some hospital settings have a regular community meeting in which both staff and patients meet together. While such a group structure is generally used for patients and staff to raise issues of concern to the community, sometimes it has been utilized as an arena in which to study the predominant emotional attitudes among the patients at a given time (Kernberg, 1984). Such meetings are deliberately less structured and thus stimulate regressive and strong sentiments. Patients may become volatile, silent, sullen, or withdrawn. Usually one particular staff member leads the meeting and may interpret important themes that emerge. Staff meet together after the meeting to share their reactions and "to diagnose" the major emotional issues that seem to be surfacing among the patients.

When group therapy itself is used as an adjunct to individual psychotherapy, the issue of whether or not the individual therapist should also lead or co-lead the group sometimes comes up. There are no hard-and-fast rules about this, unless one takes the traditional view that the transference between the patient and individual therapist should not be contaminated by the patient's experience of the therapist in group therapy. Even this argument is questionable, however, in a hospital setting in which the patients have more contact with the primary therapist and his or her other patients than would be true in an out-patient treatment. Since the therapist knows the patients individually, having them in a group may help the patients feel safe and may facilitate the work. Using a separate group therapist may provide another arena in which splitting can occur. Yet, the presence of the therapist in both individual and group modalities may be too much of a burden for both patient and therapist. It can give rise to acting-out individual transference issues in the group setting and can dilute the individual treatment. This arrangement usually works best when the patient and therapist have a stable alliance, the patient's ego functioning is somewhat more intact, and the group is for a specific purpose that complements rather than duplicates the individual treatment.

Other Adjunct Therapies

An important role of hospital treatment is to help patients to develop the skills that will enable them to function more autonomously in the community. Because borderline individuals tend to have areas of more intact or conflict-free ego functioning than is often the case with schizophrenic patients, sometimes the erroneous assumption is made that they do not need to work on improving their social and occupational skills. While vocational and other types of rehabilitative services may not be necessary for all borderline patients, they are essential for many of them. The hospital environment can provide opportunities for borderline patients to participate in activities and special training programs in which they can learn to express themselves, to socialize, to collaborate with others, to improve their interpersonal functioning, and to enhance their employability. Moreover, in the case of adolescents, educational programs often are an important component of the hospitalization. Activities and other adjunct services should be decided upon as part of the overall treatment plan and should be meaningful. Sometimes, because of their more peripheral positions in hospitals, teachers and rehabilitation therapists have important information about a patient's functioning that is not shared with others. Those staff who are involved should be integrated into the setting. This requires mechanisms for them to provide input and to receive feedback from other members of the treatment team.

Psychotropic Drugs

Until recently, the usual practice was to avoid giving medication to borderline patients. Psychotropic drugs seemed to be contraindicated both because they did not work and often were abused. With increasing interest in the relationship between borderline conditions and affective disorders, psychotic vulnerability and symptoms, severe anxiety and panic states, and other target symptoms, the selected use of medication with certain borderline patients is being advocated, particularly by those clinicians who adhere to a biological model. The literature and research on this topic is still in its infancy and the results of studies that have been conducted are unclear about the benefits of this approach. Consequently, indications for the use of drugs are vague. Often treatment response is the clearest criteria. If a patient has certain target symptoms, such as severe anxiety or depression, the patient may be given either antianxiety or antidepressant medications. If the drugs seem to relieve symptoms or suffering, enhance thinking processes and ego organization, or improve accessibility to psychotherapy, then they are considered to be effective and desirable. Another rule of thumb in using psychotropic drugs is to give antidepressants if an affective disorder seems to be present as part of or in addition to borderline personality disorder, and to administer major tranquilizers if border-line patients have pathology that is close to the psychotic range of symptoms.

Despite the potential benefits of medication, there are many problems associated with its use in borderline individuals. Minor tranquilizers relieve anxiety but generally are misused. Major tranquil-izers, while not abused and sometimes helpful in small doses, often have serious side affects. Antidepressants are highly lethal when used as part of a suicide attempt. Lithium is quite toxic when combined with alcohol. Non-compliance with drug regimens as well as abuse are common as the patient's use of medication varies with his or her attidude toward the therapist. Thus, borderline patients tend to use drugs in the acting-out of their intense and negative transference reactions. Drugs generally have positive or negative meanings to patients that go beyond their specific utility. They can be seen as an unwanted intrusion, a transitional object, a gift or sign of the therapist's caring, a magical substance that instills hope, or an indication that the therapist is giving up hope, in which case they become evidence of failure. For these reasons some clinicians separate the administration of the drug from the psychotherapy. This can reduce or eliminate their becoming involved in the transference and used for the purposes of acting-out. This practice runs the risk of increasing splitting between the psychotherapist and drug administrator. It requires close collaboration, a clear delineation of roles, and a sound understanding of borderline pathology.

DISCHARGE PLANNING

Discharge planning is an extremely important and sometimes neglected part of a long-term hospital treatment program. It requires creativity, excellent advocacy and systems negotiaion skills, and persistence on the part of those responsible for this aspect of the treatment. Even after a successful course of treatment, many borderline individuals still require follow-up care. In many instances this may involve psychotherapy only, but in some situations considerable attention to structuring the external environment in ways that resemble the positive features of the hospital environment may be necessary. Often patients will need help arranging their living situations, obtaining financial resources and other entitlements, gaining admission to special educational or job training programs, and establishing linkages to other community supports. Continuing family therapy may be indicated. The different aspects of the discharge plan need to be coordinated. In some cases, where hospitalization has not been successful in modifying destructive or highly regressive behavior, or when discharge occurs before treatment goals have been reached, patients may need to be transfered to another residential facility or may require extensive supports in order to function in the community.

Discharge planning should generally be an active, on-going part of hospital treatment from the earliest stages, rather than postponed to the termination phase or last minute. While it may not be possible or desirable to work toward the implementation of a specific discharge plan until a later point in the treatment, it is important to discuss potential options from the beginning and to maintain a balanced focus on the post-hospital period. Often patients, families, and mental health professionals themselves may be unrealistic about the outcome of treatment and do not anticipate adequately what steps may be necessary after hospitalization. An optimal discharge plan also may require a considerable amount of lead time for research on and application to various services and facilities.

Patients and families need to participate in the discharge-planning process. Much of the ground-work can be done by family members. Linkages to new therapists or programs generally should be made prior to the time the patient leaves the hospital. There should be ample time to discuss the patient's and family's reactions to the plan and specific services.

SHORT-TERM TREATMENT PRINCIPLES

Structure and Limits

Since borderline patients are typically admitted to hospitals at times of crisis, when they are extremely agitated, impulsive, or disorganized, the short-term model tends to emphasize the control function of the setting (Nurnberg & Suh, 1978). It tries to limit disruptive behavior by maintaining a firm, highly structured, unified, and predictable atmosphere in which patients must meet all rules and expectations irrespective of their pathology. While avoiding punitive interactions with patients, the staff nevertheless are encouraged to be rather strict. While aspects of this approach are useful in enabling patients to contain their behavior, it is important for staff not to behave mechanically, but to stay connected with why borderline patients become so stressed. The staff's ability to relate empathically to rather than distance themselves from patients' panic and aloneness is important in calming them and helping them to restore their inner controls.

Partialized Goals

In keeping with the need to resolve the immediate crisis that has led to the hospitalization, treatment must be partialized in its goals. It must focus on helping patients to improve those aspects of their functioning that will enable them to sustain themselves in the community. For example, if the patient's impulsiveness is a key issue, the treatment should be directed at identifying what is stimulating the patient's increased acting-out, helping the patient regain some control, modifying the internal or external conditions that may be aggravating the patient and/or enabling the patient to develop better coping mechanisms, and creating supports in the environment that can help the patient to maintain control.

Emphasis on Reality or Dynamic Issues

While the short-term nature of the treatment usually dictates that the psychotherapy engage the patient's observing ego in looking at his or her situation and how to improve it, it is important that therapists understand the varying dynamics common to borderline conditions. This can enable the therapist to arrive at meaningful speculations regarding the dynamic meaning to the patient of the events that have triggered an escalation of the patient's difficulties. In conveying this understanding to the patient, the therapist can empathically relate to what the patient is feeling and relieve some of the patient's distress. In turn, this will enable the patient to problem solve more effectively.

Confrontation or Empathy

While the therapist and staff have to mobilize the patient's motivation and positive transference in order to be of maximal help in a short-term treatment model, it may be necessary to deal with negativistic or angry behavior and responses as well as seeming indifference. Confrontation of primitive defenses and negative transference have often been stressed. Often, little attention is paid to the chronically frustrated selfobject needs, abandonment fears, panic, and hopelessness that many borderline patients feel, and which result in their provocative and "resistant" behavior. Attuned understanding of their subjective states, rather than confrontation, can be effective in reducing many of their dysfunctional responses.

A Total Approach

The psychotherapy and the hospital milieu must be coordinated. Moreover, the family must be involved in the treatment from the beginning, not only as part of the problem but as part of the solution. Medication for target symptoms may be utilized as part of a holistic approach to the patient's difficulties. The discharge plan is equally if not more important than the actual hospital treatment since it is the patient's day-to-day functioning that is so problematic. Creating and implementing a discharge plan is a key element in the hospital phase. Hopefully the hospital staff can connect patient and family to the necessary treatment and support systems that will enable the patient to attain a higher level of functioning. Often the difference between whether or not borderline patients are able to remain in the community is the degree to which the out-patient environment is structured to maintain their ego functioning while they receive psychotherapy that has more ambitious goals. While there may not be sufficient time to effect all of these arrangements, it is important to educate the patient and family in the rationale for specific recommendations and to discuss these with them in depth in the hope that they will follow through. At the very least, short-term hospitalizations should provide a positive experience to a patient and family who will need further help from professionals.

CONCLUSION

This chapter has discussed the rationale and principles of both long- and short-term hospital treatment of borderline individuals. It has described the nature of the therapeutic milieu, the treatment structure, the relationship to the family and community, treatment modalities, discharge planning, and short-term treatment techniques. While clinical experience seems to suggest that a range of treatment options is desirable, mental health care policy and funding in the United States favor acute rather than long-term in-patient care. Length of stay generally is a function of the nature of patients' insurance rather than their clinical condition. While it is important to improve the short-term hospital treatment phase by experimenting with new approaches and providing quality care, the treatment of borderline pathology usually requires long-term aftercare in the community or repeated hospitalizations. The lack of long-term in-patient settings is compounded by the absence of follow-up care in the community that is suited to the special needs of borderline patients. Thus, individuals who can be helped are deprived of both in- and out-patient services. The situation is grim and not getting better. It is important that practitioners of a variety of mental health disciplines join with consumers in working for an improvement in the organization and delivery of mental health services.

10

Couple and Family Treatment

In work with borderline individuals there are many instances in which the treatment of the family system is necessary for therapeutic success. The therapist's failure to understand and treat interlocking interpersonal pathology in couples and families may result in therapeutic impasses. Sometimes a couple or family will present with an "identified" borderline member as is generally the case when hospitalization is involved, while in out-patient treatment and private practice clinicians will encounter "borderline" couples or families—that is, families in which there is at least one borderline member. Couple or family therapy is indicated in those cases in which current interpersonal transactions seem to be aggravating or perpetuating the problems of the identified borderline patient, or in which there is shared couple or family pathology that weakens the system's functioning. In many cases conjoint couple or family therapy (as contrasted with the simultaneous individual treatment of different family members) may be the main treatment modality. This frequently accompanies individual psychotherapy.

While numerous couple and family treatment models have been put forth, object-relations and self psychological approaches are most consistent with the developmental perspectives on borderline disorders that have been discussed in this volume. While conceptually distinct, they each focus on: (1) understanding the impact of past developmental needs and arrests on current interpersonal transactions; (2) the individual within the couple and family as well as the family as a system;

(3) developing insight into dysfunctional patterns of interaction; and (4) altering developmental difficulties as well as current behavior. Both approaches require that family members possess a certain degree of verbal facility, observing ego, and self-differentiation.

The main differences between the object-relations and self psychological approaches are reflected in the attention the former model gives to the interpretation of how primitive defenses and internalized object relations affect couple and family interactions, in contrast to the prominence the latter model gives to the identification of selfobject needs and what frustrates them, and the interpretation of the impact of past parental selfobject failures on interpersonal interactions. While some clinicians might argue that a distinguishing feature of the self psychological model is its systematic use of a subjective and empathic approach, many object-relations family therapists rely heavily on the use of empathy in providing a therapeutic holding environment. I do agree, however, that the object-relations model is less experience-near than is the self psychological model. This chapter will present and illustrate the application of both object-relations and self psychological principles and techniques to couple and family therapy with borderline individuals.

ADVANTAGES OF CONJOINT COUPLE AND FAMILY TREATMENT

In conjoint couple or family treatment family members are seen together by one or more therapists. Individual sessions may also be used selectively or on a regular basis with each participant, or another therapist may see family members on an individual basis. There are numerous advantages to conjoint treatment in work with borderline individuals. When there is an identified borderline patient, pathological family interactions can be identified and ameliorated, and the identified borderline patient's perceptions of family interactions can be validated. Helping the borderline patient to receive an understanding of the power of pathological family transactions can assist him or her to separate from the family. At times, having the patient observe the shared and collusive nature of the pathology can also have positive effects. Transferences are already manifest in the couple or family interactions and do not need to be created in the therapeutic relationship. These primitive transferences and distortions are often less intense and more accessible to modification in family sessions. The therapist is better able to provide a holding environment for each family member and to point out dysfunctional interactions without seeming to blame or criticize. Further, the egocentric perspectives of individual family members can be broadened so that they become more empathic with one another.

AN OBJECT-RELATIONS MODEL

An object-relations treatment model with couples and families views past family interactions as having become internalized by each family member. This leads to distortions of current interpersonal transactions and to repetitive and dysfunctional patterns of relating. As discussed in Chapter 5, object-relations family theorists generally view the defenses of splitting, denial, and projective identification as common to border-line couples and families. They also point to their conflicts around intimacy, autonomy and dependence, and fears of abandonment and rejection.

Goals

Object-relations couple and family therapy aims at both helping members of a couple or family to perceive and relate to one another in terms of their "here and now" qualities rather than as representatives of their troubled, internalized, past significant relationships, and at expanding the family's capacity to differentiate, to nurture, and to support the autonomy of its members. The therapist works both with current interactions and past developmental and family-of-origin is-sues. Depending on their theoretical leanings, the object-relations family therapists differ to some degree in their emphasis. For example, Scharff and Scharff (1987) focus on helping family members to understand their difficulties in providing "good enough holding" for one another and to improve their "holding" capacities. In contrast, Slipp (1988) and Stewart et al. (1975) put more stress on the identifi-cation and modification of the primitive defenses of splitting and projective identification, and on the collusive patterns that dominate couple and family interactions.

Major Principles

Developing a Holding Environment

Borderline couples and families who seek treatment are often locked into intense and acrimonious interactions that stem from their primi-tive defenses; demandingness; unpredictability; fears of closeness;

sensitivity to criticism and rejection; separation and abandonment fears; competitiveness for nurturing; low self-esteem; angry outbursts and impulsiveness; violence and self-destructive behavior; boundary difficulties; and potential for fragmentation. From the very beginning of treatment a safe and consistent therapeutic climate must be created for all family members. The therapist does this by providing a clear and firm structure, with boundaries against destructive acting-out, and by showing acceptance, promoting trust, lowering defensiveness, tolerating intense and unpleasant affects, facilitating communication and mutual empathy, and containing aggression so as not to permit excessive blaming, scapegoating, or loss of control. The therapist must refrain from countertransference acting-out, particularly with respect to power struggles and counteraggression and should be genuine and nonexploitative, self-observant and self-controlled, and honest about errors or possibly insensitive comments. Efforts to establish a holding environment are illustrated in the two examples presented below.

In the case of Debbie and her psychiatrist parents, the Fines, who were described in Chapter 5, family sessions were undertaken to diffuse the family system's scapegoating of Debbie and to foster family members' ability to relate to one another in more realistic and individualized ways. Both parents presented themselves as strong and independent. They regarded Debbie as weak, emotional, and dependent, and devalued and rejected her. Depressed and suicidal, Debbie regarded herself as inadequate and a failure, and idealized her parents. In early family sessions her parents harangued Debbie verbally and attempted to get the therapist to ally with them. Debbie became increasingly more withdrawn and self-disparaging. Instead of expressing her feelings or asserting herself, she seemed to look to the therapist to defend or rescue her. Her attitude and demeanor led to an escalation of the parents' accusations. In numerous sessions the therapist repeatedly intervened by setting a limit on the expression of negative feelings, empathically relating to the pain each family member was feeling, reframing the problem as one the family faced together, and defining her role as being supportive of the whole family.

MOTHER: I can't understand how you can just sit there and not try to help yourself. We don't see you doing anything to cooperate with the treatment. We're tired of watching you destroy yourself and us in the process.

DEBBIE: I think you should just give up on me. I know I'm hurting you.

FATHER: Then why do you let yourself vegetate? Why don't you pull yourself up by the bootstraps? You've never shown any fight. I don't know what's wrong with you.

DEBBIE: I'm always going to be a disappointment to you.

FATHER: I can't go on shelling out money for your treatment if you aren't going to make an effort. I have many patients who haven't had the opportunities that we've given you.

THERAPIST: It must be very hard to see Debbie so depressed and immobilized.

MOTHER: She doesn't seem to want to help herself.

THERAPIST: I can see how angry and frustrated both you and your husband are feeling but continuing to vent your anger at Debbie is not going to help us all to better understand what will help the family.

MOTHER: We are not angry people. Debbie provokes us to lose control.

FATHER: My wife and I both are used to dealing with sick people but Debbie doesn't want to cooperate with us — Debbie, are you listening to me or more interested in staring at the wall?

DEBBIE: I am listening to you.

MOTHER: You don't act like it!

THERAPIST: I know that both of you are trying your best to reach Debbie, but I am going to have to ask you to try to contain your angry outbursts at her. This is a very difficult time for everyone in the family.

MOTHER: Debbie is the one with the problems. My husband and I have done our best and no one helped us I can tell you.

THERAPIST: I see three people here who are in pain, not just one. Each of you has an investment in our trying to find a better solution. What all of you have been doing together isn't working. I am going to try to help all of you work this out.

FATHER: What do you suggest?

In the case of Dave and Barbara, who came for help to save their marriage, early sessions were so volatile and mutually accusatory that each partner threatened to leave the office. While the therapist felt it was important to tolerate their highly charged interactions to a degree, it became clear that the couple was unable to move beyond their fighting. The therapist intervened by pointing out how stuck the couple was in their mutually hurtful battles and setting a limit on their fighting. She was able to relate empathically to what each member of the couple was feeling, and actively structure their interaction to be more productive.

DAVE: You are a controlling bitch!

BARBARA: Mr. Control himself is talking. You're such a hypocrite. You can't see what a Hitler you are.

DAVE: I'm going to hit you, I swear.

BARBARA: Go ahead. You're such an animal.

THERAPIST: Let's stop a minute and look at what's happening. You are both so angry that it seems impossible for you to talk without your both trying to destroy one another.

DAVE: Barbara just won't listen to me.

BARBARA: I won't listen to you? You are such an asshole!

THERAPIST: I know that each of you feels justified in your accusations, but by continuing to attack one another you can't get beyond your anger. This is where the two of you are stuck. We have to focus on helping you to hear one another.

BARBARA: I don't think Dave ever thinks that I have feelings.

DAVE: You. . . .

THERAPIST: Wait a minute, Dave. What do you hear Barbara saying?

DAVE: That I'm inhuman.

BARBARA: You're . . . .

THERAPIST: Wait a minute, Barbara.

BARBARA: Okay. Okay. I'm sorry.

THERAPIST: I know you feel attacked when Barbara says something like that to you and you want to get back at her.

DAVE: Yes. I don't know why she says that about me.

THERAPIST: Is it possible for you to try to find out what she is experiencing?

BARBARA: He doesn't know how to listen.

THERAPIST: Barbara, you too have trouble refraining from attacking Dave. It just happened right here. Could you try telling Dave what you are feeling without accusing him or defending yourself?

BARBARA: He just makes me so angry.

THERAPIST: You both have that affect on each other at this point. We need to find a way for you to talk to and hear each other better without tearing each other apart.

DAVE: How?

THERAPIST: We need to make this a space where you both can learn to express what you are feeling without fearing that you are going to be attacked or judged. It's important that each of you try to hear what the other is saying.

Identifying Dysfunctional Interactions and Sequences

As members of a troubled couple or family interact in sessions the therapist is in an optimal position to observe the ways in which they are unable to support and provide "holding" for one another; how they perceive and relate in distorted ways; and how repetitive, rigid, and destructive their behavioral sequences are. The therapist's ability to interrupt and point out dysfunctional behavior requires an active but non-blaming stance. This necessity of providing a safe environment that limits destructive behavior and points out dysfunctional interactions without jeopardizing individual members' experience of the therapist as empathic is one of the most difficult challenges of this approach.

In early family sessions with the Fines it soon became evident that when Debbie talked about her fears of abandonment, sadness, or low self-esteem, both parents responded with a lecture about how she should be doing more to help herself rather than with any empathic exploration of or reaction to Debbie's feelings. Instead of showing her anger and demanding to be heard, Debbie clammed up, thereby reinforcing her parents' view of her as dependent, inadequate, and uncaring. In a non-blaming tone the therapist drew attention to this collusive pattern of interaction and to the family's difficulty in relating more positively to one another.

DEBBIE: I've been feeling so badly lately. I don't know what to do. I feel defeated.

FATHER: That's just another example of how negative you are.

MOTHER: I don't see why you can't think more positively.

DEBBIE: It's no use.

MOTHER: You always say that. I don't know what to say to you.

THERAPIST: It seems to be very hard to talk about sad feelings in the family.

FATHER: What do you mean?

THERAPIST: When Debbie spoke of her sadness and despair, it was difficult for both of you to hear what she was saying and to ask her more about herself. Instead you gave her a well-intentioned lecture that Debbie experienced as your not really hearing her.

MOTHER: We just want to help.

THERAPIST: I can see how hard you both try. When Debbie doesn't respond positively and looks more depressed, you get frustrated rather than ask her what she needs. Debbie, you give up instead of letting your parents know what they're doing to upset you. You withdraw and seem not to care. You feel more alone and they feel more helpless and frustrated.

MOTHER: How can we break the pattern?

The therapist made a similar intervention with Barbara and Dave when they revealed a repetitive pattern of using anger to create distance between them.

BARBARA: Since we've been coming for therapy, I'm feeling a little closer to Dave.

DAVE: I want to bring something up. Why didn't you pay the bills yesterday? You say you want to participate more in our financial affairs and then you don't follow through.

BARBARA: I had to take care of our daughter while you were out playing racquetball with your friends.

DAVE: I'm entitled to some fun. You're a slave driver.

THERAPIST: Let's stop a minute and look at what just happened to make you both start attacking each other.

BARBARA: I'm really angry. I take a risk and show my positive feelings for you and what do you do? You've got to remind me that I'm an irresponsible child.

THERAPIST: How did Barbara's comment about feeling closer to you make you feel?

DAVE: I don't know. I guess I pushed her away. It's not all me. Barbara, what did you do when I came over to hug you yesterday? *You* pushed *me* away and in an ugly voice told me my timing was terrible, as if I had the plague or something.

BARBARA: I don't like your trying to get close to me when I'm fixing dinner. Maybe I was nasty. It's a reflex action.

THERAPIST: When one of you comes closer, the other makes an angry comment that is distancing and you perpetuate your conflict. Perhaps you are both frightened of getting closer?

Improving the Family's Holding Function

The therapist goes beyond pointing out the family's inability or difficulties in supporting one another and actively tries to foster more optimal "holding" through suggestion and example. Many borderline families literally do not know how to communicate positively, effectively, and lovingly. Thus, the therapist uses himself or herself in the therapeutic interaction to create and demonstrate more optimal ways of relating, as is shown in the following vignettes.

DEBBIE: I get so lonely and scared sometimes.

FATHER: Don't you have people around whom you can go to?

DEBBIE: I feel too depressed.

FATHER: You have to make yourself reach out to other people.

THERAPIST: I'm going to interrupt here. This is another example of what happens when Debbie starts to share her feelings. I can see you and your wife getting agitated and Debbie withdrawing. Maybe you could share what you felt when Debbie said she was lonely and scared.

FATHER: I guess I just get frightened myself that she's never going to get better and I feel helpless. I want her to get better. I think my wife feels the same way.

THERAPIST: Is your husband right?

MOTHER: I don't know if I feel helpless. I think I feel more depressed and confused. I don't know how this could have happened.

THERAPIST: So it seems that when Debbie expresses herself, both of you begin to feel sad and start questioning yourselves. It's hard for you to stay with what Debbie is experiencing without trying to fix her. Perhaps it would be better if you could just tell Debbie how you are feeling?

MOTHER: I don't want to see you suffer. I want to help. Doesn't it come through?

DEBBIE: I feel like a bad person when you lecture me and I feel that I'd be better off dead.

THERAPIST: It must be painful to hear Debbie say that.

FATHER: I feel upset and a little hopeless.

MOTHER: I do too.

THERAPIST: I know it is hard for both of you to feel that way. You try to get away from these feelings by fixing Debbie. Unfortunately, Debbie then feels angry and expresses her anger by becoming more depressed. It's a vicious cycle. Perhaps you could try to draw Debbie out more about what she is feeling and why?

With Dave and Barbara the therapist similarly tried to help them to be more responsive to one another.

BARBARA: I would like Dave to show more affection.

DAVE: Every time I try to do that you reject me.

BARBARA: That's not true.

THERAPIST: What happened when Barbara said she wanted you to show her more affection?

DAVE: I felt she was accusing me of being cold.

THERAPIST: That felt unfair?

DAVE: Yes.

THERAPIST: When you feel that way it is hard for you to find out more about what she wants and needs. Instead, you get caught up in feeling attacked and want to fight back.

DAVE: It's her nasty tone of voice.

THERAPIST: So you don't feel much like drawing her out at that point?

BARBARA: Maybe sometimes I do have an attitude that comes through, but not always. I think Dave hears me a certain way no matter how I talk to him.

DAVE: She may be right. I think I know what she's going to say before she says it.

THERAPIST: You seem to be able to hear one another right now. That's important. Maybe we could get back to what Barbara said about wanting you to show her affection. Are you sure you know what it is that she wants?

DAVE: She wants me to make love to her more often.

BARBARA: I would like that, but that's not what I mean by wanting you to show me affection.

DAVE: What do you mean?

BARBARA: I'd like you to come over to me sometimes and just show me that you care without wanting sex.

DAVE: I never know when you are going to reject me.

Interpreting Primitive Defenses

The presence of primitive defenses and collusive processes create distorted perceptions and interactions within the family context. Frustration and intense rage result when different partners feel that they are being viewed in a rigid, stereotyped fashion that does not really portray who they are. Because of the unconscious nature of denial and splitting, each member does not have an accurate perception of the provocative ways he or she behaves. A major therapeutic intervention in work with borderline couples and families is the interpretation of splitting, denial, and projective identification, as well as of the ways in which each family member participates in pathological transactions. The therapist helps parents or members of a couple to accept traits and feelings in themselves that they have denied, disavowed, and projected onto one another, and to lessen their distortions of one another. Thus, the treatment fosters differentiation. Modifying the family's characteristic patterns of defenses in this manner takes time and is based on the therapist's understanding of the individual personalities and developmental histories of the couple or family, as well as their current interaction.

In the Fine family, denial, splitting, and projective identification were reflected in the parents' sense of strength and perfection, which they equated with "goodness," and their repudiation of their own feelings of weakness, dependence, and emotionality, which they equated with "badness." Their son possessed all the "good" qualities and Debbie embodied the "bad" characteristics. They saw their own unfavorable and disavowed traits in her. In turn, Debbie complied with their projections and devalued herself while idealizing them. In family sessions the therapist tried to help the parents to acknowledge those feelings in themselves that they denied and to lessen their rigid view of Debbie.

FATHER: I can't stand it when Debbie acts helpless and clings to us. I want her to be more independent.

MOTHER: Our son is totally different from Debbie. He's more like us. Debbie has always been different.

THERAPIST: I guess I'm struck by the fact that both you and your husband seem to see yourselves as totally independent and strong people who are in control of your emotions and see Debbie as the exact opposite.

FATHER: That's how Debbie is.

THERAPIST: Both of you seem to feel that being dependent is a weakness. You both have tried so hard in your own lives to be independent people.

FATHER: If I hadn't, I never would have survived.

MOTHER: I can't bear to think about what would have happened to me if I hadn't done for myself. There was no one there to take care of me.

THERAPIST: Both of you were neglected as children. It's remarkable what you have done in your lives. I think it's very painful for you to relate emotionally to how bad it was for you back then.

FATHER: I don't want to look back.

MOTHER: We are optimistic people. We look ahead.

THERAPIST: Perhaps Debbie's problems make you reexperience painful feelings that belong to your childhoods?

DEBBIE: I didn't know that you had such a hard time when you were younger. Why haven't you ever talked about it?

MOTHER: I'd rather forget. It's all in the past. I get angry at you sometimes because I didn't have the help from my parents that you get from us.

THERAPIST: You want Debbie to be independent in the way that you and your husband are.

MOTHER: Yes.

THERAPIST: Is it possible that sometimes you stress that too much?

FATHER: I'm not sure what you mean.

THERAPIST: It seems so important to both of you that Debbie be independent, and not remind you of the pain of being helpless and depressed, that you have trouble listening to Debbie and accepting her as she is.

MOTHER: I don't know how she could be so different from us.

THERAPIST: I'm suggesting that she's not so different from the way you once were.

MOTHER: There may be some truth in that. It makes me very sad to think about this.

THERAPIST: I know it is difficult but we have to look at some of these issues in order to free all of you.

Dave and Barbara also evidenced denial, splitting, and projective identification in the ways in which they accused each other of being childish, irresponsible, controlling, and angry, while refusing to acknowledge these traits in themselves. They alternately assumed the roles of parent and child with one another. The therapist attempted to make them aware of their distortions and characteristic patterns of relating.

BARBARA: I can't stand it when you treat me like a child!

DAVE: Then don't be irresponsible. Act your age!

BARBARA: Don't lay a trip on me! You don't always act so adult yourself. You love being a little boy.

THERAPIST: Both of you are name-calling again. You each accuse the other of acting like a child and being irresponsible, but don't seem to realize how you mutually provoke one another. When Barbara does things that you think are infantile you, Dave, come on like a parent trying to discipline a "bad" child, and when Dave acts in ways that you, Barbara, think are irresponsible, you become the harsh parent.

BARBARA: That sounds like us.

THERAPIST: I know that both of you feel that your reactions are totally justified. You manage unwittingly to provoke the other into playing out the critical parent when you become the irresponsible child. Your relationship begins to feel like it is repeating your worst childhood experiences.

DAVE: Maybe we're not cut out to be with one another.

THERAPIST: That's not necessarily true. I think that you can learn to relate to each other differently and see one another more realistically.

Separating Past from Present

In couple and family therapy with borderline individuals family members display intense transference reactions with one another that distort the interpersonal field and replay early relationships with parents and significant others. Parents and members of a couple, in particular, often experience themselves as children in relation to parental figures with whom they are locked in verbal battles, mutual victimization, and sometimes outright abuse and violence. Thus, past experience that has become internalized colors current perceptions and interactions, even though family members actually may be acting in keeping with the roles they are being assigned. The therapist identifies the transferential component in certain reactions by connecting them to past family-of-origin experiences. Treatment focuses on separating the present from the past in order to free family members to interact with

one another in terms of their "real" rather than transferential characteristics. Sometimes family members feel that interventions of this type
minimize what they are experiencing in the present and point out
evidence for why their husband or wife, for example, really does
resemble a parental figure. Because there is a kernel of truth to their
perceptions, they have difficulty accepting that they are "overreacting"
because of past experiences.

BARBARA: Don't all couples fight like this?

THERAPIST: I don't think you are just fighting with each other, in
regard to what is taking place currently. You are also replaying issues
from your own past that make it hard to see each other realistically.

DAVE: I can't stand it when Barbara acts like my mother.

BARBARA: That's a laugh. Most of the time you tell me I'm
behaving like a child and you treat me the way your mother treats you.

DAVE: You really can't look at yourself, Barbara.

THERAPIST: You both are bringing your past experiences with you
into the relationship and playing out what is familiar to you, even
though it's painful. You don't realize how both of you provoke one
another to play out the role of a critical parent, whom you loved and
hated at the same time. It feels real. You experience the intense feelings
now that you did when you were children.

BARBARA: What can we do to stop it?

THERAPIST: The first step is to begin to tell yourselves that this is
what is happening when you start escalating, and to then try to stop and
listen to one another's needs.

Working Through Negative Introjects and Internalized
Object Relations

In many instances it is important to go beyond the interpretation of
primitive defenses and transference reactions to help individual members of a couple or family to identify and let go of their negative
introjects and internalized self- and object-relations. This can be
accomplished in conjoint sessions, usually in conjunction with some
individual work, but working through this process may take a long
time. For example, both Dave and Barbara had deep fears about being
unlovable and of being abandoned, both of which stemmed from their
early lives. Even when either partner acted in more caring and
affectionate ways, the other would find a way of distancing or
otherwise sabotaging the interaction. In addition to making them aware
of how they contributed to the closeness–distancing pattern, the
therapist worked at length with each of them on identifying and

ameliorating the negative self- and object-representations that were dominating their current self concepts and close relationships.

Using Countertransference

During the treatment process the therapist becomes the object of transference and primitive defenses which, because of their intense nature, stimulate strong feelings, or what has been termed "induced countertransference," in the therapist. As discussed in Chapter 6, this refers both to understandable reactions the therapist has to the patient's extreme behavior and to the therapist's identification with the patient's disavowed and projected inner feelings or objects or internalized self- and object-relationships. Induced countertransference reactions tell the therapist a great deal about the nature of the internalized self- and object-representations that manifest in transferences with family members and the therapist. Thus, couple or family therapists must recognize and understand their countertransference reactions and use this understanding in their interventions to help the couple or parents understand their inner world, past experiences, and how these play out in the here-and-now of family life.

After a period of seemingly productive work with Dave and Barbara, they canceled their next two sessions. When they came for their next scheduled appointment they did not communicate freely with one another but did not seem to mind. When the therapist explored this the couple became antagonistic to the therapist, who found herself feeling rejected and mildly irritated. The therapist recognized that Dave and Barbara were enacting their closeness–distancing pattern with her and tried to address this dynamic.

THERAPIST: Neither of you seem to have much to say today.

DAVE: Do we have to always analyze everything?

BARBARA: We need a rest.

THERAPIST: Is that why you canceled your last two appointments?

BARBARA: We couldn't get a babysitter. Our regular one is busy.

THERAPIST: How have you been getting along?

DAVE: Nothing's new.

THERAPIST: I'm a little puzzled by what's happening tonight. The last time we were together you seemed to be very involved in working on your relationship and expressed feelings that you were making progress. Since then you have been unable to make it to your sessions and tonight you are saying you both want a rest.

DAVE: It was good to have some time off.

BARBARA: I hardly noticed that we weren't here.

THERAPIST: I wonder if you're feeling angry with me.

BARBARA: You're reading too much into it.

THERAPIST: We've talked in the past about how you each begin to distance from one another when the other approaches in a more positive way. I wonder if something like that is happening between the two of you and me. Perhaps you were feeling more trusting of me and opening up more, and now you are both distancing in order to protect yourselves?

BARBARA: Sometimes I do wonder when you are going to lower the boom on me.

THERAPIST: What do you mean by lowering the boom?

BARBARA: You always seem very accepting, even when I act like a bratty kid. I think you are going to get tired of me or angry or something.

DAVE: Now that we're talking about this, I remember wondering what you thought of what I told you the last session about my mother having beat me when I was younger.

THERAPIST: What were you concerned about?

DAVE: I thought maybe you thought I deserved it or that I was bad-mouthing my parents.

THERAPIST: Each of you experience a lot of anxiety when you let down your defenses. You become afraid that you are vulnerable and can possibly be hurt. You each begin to experience yourselves as victimized children, in relation to others who become critical and attacking parental figures. Sometimes you act in ways that bring on the behavior you fear. You do this with one another and it is now coming up in our relationship too.

BARBARA: I'm beginning to see that pattern more clearly.

A SELF PSYCHOLOGICAL MODEL

A self psychological treatment model views couple and family problems as reflecting individual deficits in intrapsychic structure that result in the expression and mutual frustration of archaic selfobject needs (for example, for mirroring, idealization, and twinship). As discussed in Chapter 5, borderline and narcissistic parents look to one another and their offspring to compensate for their self deficits in the maintenance of self-esteem and self-cohesion. When selfobject needs are frustrated, defensive and dysfunctional patterns of interaction ensue (Lachkar, 1985; Magdoff & Greenberg, 1988; Solomon, 1985).

Goals

In applying self psychological principles as discussed in Chapter 7 to the treatment of couples and families one aims at identifying and fostering empathy for each family member's selfobject needs, pointing out how they are being repetitively frustrated, and, ultimately, at promoting greater fulfillment of each family member's selfobject needs. The therapist not only addresses here-and-now interactions, but also helps family members to understand the developmental origins of their selfobject needs, the defenses against them, and the rage and depletion states that ensue when selfobject needs are frustrated.

Major Principles

Empathizing with Each Member of the Couple or Family

The bedrock of a self psychological approach is the therapist's ability to be attuned to each family member's subjective experience through empathic immersion. He or she must also be able to acknowledge their individual and sometimes conflicting selfobject needs, and, in some instances, to function as a selfobject (White, 1984). This requires that the therapist abandon a neutral position in the traditional sense because neutrality is not experienced as empathic but rather as uninvolved and objective. The task for the therapist is to distribute his or her empathy equally. The therapist's empathic attunement to each family member's needs, thoughts, and feelings helps them to feel accepted and understood, to be more open in sharing feelings, and to be more able to listen to and hear one another.

While the therapist's provision of empathy is not to be equated with agreement, it still poses problems, such as the attempt to be empathic with different members of the same family in the same space at the same time. Certain individuals may become upset if the therapist seems too understanding or supportive of another family member, or when the therapist is empathic with someone who has conflicting needs or polarized perceptions. Finding the proper balance between too little and too much responsiveness, and helping each person in the family feel validated without taking sides, are major therapeutic tasks. This is especially difficult with borderline patients who are so extreme, needy of affirmation, competitive for nurturing, and volatile.

In the case of Angela and Mark, which was described in Chapter 5, each presented diametrically opposed views of their interaction, and at the same time looked to the therapist for validation. The therapist tried to be attuned to what each partner was experiencing subjectively without either agreeing or disagreeing with the "objective truth" of what was being said. This became more difficult when each partner attempted to get the therapist to take sides.

MARK: I can't take Angela's withdrawal from me. She shuts me out.

ANGELA: All you want to do is to control my every move. I need space. If you feel shut out, that's your problem.

THERAPIST: Can you tell me a little more about what makes you feel that Angela is shutting you out?

MARK: I try to ask her about her day and she won't talk to me.

ANGELA: That's not true. I tell you about my day and you want to know every detail of where I went and what I did. It's like you are sure I am lying to you and you want to catch me.

THERAPIST: You feel Mark is too possessive.

ANGELA: Yes. He calls me several times a day and if I'm not at the number where he thinks I'm going to be, he goes crazy.

MARK: I don't go crazy. Don't make me look like a madman.

THERAPIST: You seem to feel very desperate when Angela is unavailable or doesn't want to share her thoughts and feelings with you.

MARK: She doesn't appreciate that I love her and care about her. I worry if I can't reach her.

THERAPIST: I guess you feel that if she cared about you she wouldn't put you through this.

MARK: That's exactly how I feel.

ANGELA: I don't understand this. I'm at work. Where do you think I am? What is going to happen to me? I need to have some time to myself.

THERAPIST: You seem to feel that Mark is not just worried about your well-being but is trying to control you.

ANGELA: Yes! Don't you think that a man who has to know my whereabouts every minute of the day is controlling? I can't even talk on the telephone to a friend without his questioning me about the conversation. Don't you think that's a little odd?

THERAPIST: It's understandable that you feel that he is not being sensitive to your needs.

MARK: She is making me sound like a raging paranoid. I need you to tell her that it is not abnormal to be interested in someone you love.

THERAPIST: I can see that each of you feels very strongly about what you are saying, and I can understand what is making each of you feel that the other is controlling on the one hand and withholding on the other. It's difficult for each of you to understand that you may have conflicting needs at times.

Developing Empathy for Each Family Member's Selfobject Needs

Everyone has selfobject needs that manifest in different ways and may evolve and change over the course of ones life. Even when these are mature, they may result in couple and family conflict. In borderline couples and families archaic selfobject needs predominate. This indicates selfobject failures and traumas at the hands of parents and significant others in childhood. These needs feel urgent and often seem extreme. When they are frustrated, intense reactions follow. When seeking help, couples and families often have difficulty listening to and really hearing one another. This stems not only from the heightened degree of conflict and bad feelings that are present, but also because each member of a couple, for example, speaks a different emotional language, so to speak. They tend to interpret one another's behavior in terms of their own reactions, and are unable to understand or accept that a partner may have different motivations and feelings than they have themselves. Even if there is an accurate perception of the differences in the ways partners feel or behave, these dissimilarities are viewed as "wrong" or "stupid" rather than respected as understandable reflections of a unique or separate personality. An extremely important therapeutic intervention involves sensitizing family members to each other's individual needs and ways of thinking and feeling, thereby expanding their capacity for empathy with one another, as is shown in the example below.

ANGELA: Why do you get so angry when I'm just taking the space that I need?

MARK: I've told you a thousand times that I do not mind when you are occupied. I get upset when you shut me out. You do it deliberately to hurt me. You don't understand how desperate I feel.

ANGELA: What you call shutting you out is my not being available to you on command. If you get desperate, that's not my fault.

MARK: Every time that I have wanted to make love to you the last few weeks you haven't wanted to. Then when you don't want to tell me where you have been, of course I worry that you have lost interest in me.

THERAPIST: That must make you feel quite panicky.

MARK: Yes. I don't understand why Angela can't give me the reassurance that I need.

THERAPIST: It seems difficult for you to imagine that Angela's needs for privacy or to be left alone sexually at times have nothing to do with the love she feels for you.

MARK: I feel that if she loved me, she would want to be with me and confide in me.

ANGELA: I do confide in and want to be with you, but not all the time. You don't seem to appreciate what I do to show you that I care. I do everything I'm supposed to do for him. I work, clean, and make him dinner. I can't help it if I'm too tired to enjoy making love every night. He never leaves me alone.

MARK: You're making me sound like a sexual compulsive. I keep asking you because you keep saying no. I know that you work hard but don't you want to be with me?

THERAPIST: Each of you has different needs for closeness, and unfairly judge the other's actions by your own standards. When Mark frustrates your need for space you, Angela, withdraw more and this panics Mark. You, Mark, become more demanding of attention and this pushes Angela further away. It's hard for you, Angela, to accept how desperate Mark feels and to give him some reassurance that you still care for him and you, Mark, can't back off and give Angela some time to herself without feeling personally rejected.

ANGELA: Mark just doesn't understand that I'm different than he is. I have always been this way.

THERAPIST: It seems that you want Mark to be more like you just as he wants you to be more like him.

ANGELA: You have a point. I just keep feeling that he is trying to control me.

MARK: I wish you would understand that it's not about control. I just get frightened that you are interested in someone else and are going to leave me. I know I get extreme sometimes.

THERAPIST: Can you imagine that it feels controlling to Angela.

MARK: If I try to put myself in her place I guess I can see that.

Identifying Mutually Frustrating Interactions and Defenses

The repetitive lack of recognition and failure to gratify one another's selfobject needs lead to vicious cycles of mutually frustrating interactions. Further, members of a couple or family erect defenses to protect themselves from narcissistic injury and to preserve their self-esteem and self-cohesion. These defenses tend to result in conflict, power struggles, and feelings of victimization as one member of a couple, for example, withdraws in order to preserve his or her autonomy and the other provokes a fight in order to maintain contact. The therapist empathically comments on and relates to the needs underlying the dysfunctional interactions and the defensive patterns that are established.

ANGELA: We had a terrible fight over the weekend. I thought Mark was going to hit me.

MARK: She enraged me. I did lose control but I wasn't going to hurt her. She never even tries to help me calm down. She does everything possible to provoke me.

ANGELA: What you call calming you is my giving in to you. I won't do that. I'm not going to cater to your needs.

THERAPIST: Who would like to share what happened?

MARK: I want you to get an accurate picture of what occurred. I bought a new suit and I tried it on to show Angela. I thought it looked nice and I wanted her opinion. She told me that she didn't think it did anything for me and that it made me look older. I was hurt.

ANGELA: Did you want my opinion or did you just want me to tell you how handsome you looked?

MARK: I'm going to ignore that comment. Anyway, I told Angela that I was hurt and she said that it was not part of her job to have to build up my ego all the time. She looked at me with hatred, all because I asked her about my suit. I got angry but she refused to talk to me. She stormed into another room and slammed the door. I went after her and tried to talk to her and she locked the door. I banged on the door and threatened to break it down. She told me that she was going to call the police. She sounded frightened so I just left the apartment.

THERAPIST: That must have been quite upsetting for both of you.

ANGELA: Mark is only telling you half of the story. What Mark is leaving out is what happened before he put his suit on. I was on the telephone with my sister when Mark barged into the room and told me to get off the phone because he had something to show me. I told him that I don't interrupt him when he's busy. I wouldn't get off the phone and he started to pout.

MARK: I don't know why you had to speak in such an angry tone to me. What was wrong with my wanting your attention? You didn't have to yell at me?

THERAPIST: Angela wanted you to be sensitive to her need to talk to someone else privately without being interrupted. Mark needed your immediate attention. It is difficult for each of you to respect where the other is coming from without feeling personally attacked. You both feel that the other is deliberately trying to frustrate your needs and so you each feel justified in your positions. This escalates into an ongoing power struggle that makes each of you feel miserable. We have to focus on how to help you understand and meet each others' needs to a greater degree, and to cope better when some of those needs conflict and are inevitably frustrated.

ANGELA: I would like to resolve this.

THERAPIST: It is not hard to understand why you feel justifiably angry with Mark for what you experience as his insensitivity to your needs, but you must realize that you also negate some of his needs. What do you think the impact of that is on Mark?

ANGELA: I guess he feels that I don't care about him.

MARK: That's right. I don't know why you have to be so withholding. It just makes me feel and act worse.

THERAPIST: I can understand your feeling rejected, Mark, but do you suppose it makes Angela feel very loving toward you when you repeatedly seem to ignore her need for privacy and threaten her with violence?

MARK: I love her. I'm not going to hurt her.

ANGELA: You have a strange way of showing your love. It's hard to feel that you love me when you treat me that way.

MARK: I don't know how we can stop this or why it's even happening.

Linking Present Interactions to Past Selfobject Failures

The archaic selfobject needs and mutually frustrating interactions that one sees in borderline couples and families are linked directly to developmental failures in empathy on the part of parents and caretakers. Thus, current interactions are shaped by the past. The therapist interprets the connection between past and present in order to help family members understand and appreciate their own needs and behavior, to lessen the hold that developmental failures have on their relationships, and to help them find better ways of gratifying their needs.

MARK: I don't know why I get so panicky when Angela isn't responsive to me in the way that I'd like. It's almost an automatic reaction on my part.

Angela: It's interesting that you should say that. I feel the same way. I can't stop my reaction when Mark expects me to be there for him or doesn't respect the things that I need to do for myself.

THERAPIST: We've talked some about your early childhood experiences. It is understandable that some of these are influencing the way you both interact now. From what we have talked about previously, it seems that neither of you were able to rely on your parents for any kind of consistent or caring responsiveness. Mark was continually being abandoned by his mother and you, Angela, were always expected to take care of both of your parents. You weren't allowed to have any needs of your own.

ANGELA: How does that influence our relationship?

THERAPIST: Perhaps you feel fear that once again you will have to submerge your needs, this time in favor of Mark's, and maybe you, Mark, fear the abandonment that you were so accustomed to? In some ways you both expect that the past will be repeated. In other ways you hope that it will be different. Each of you needs the other to be perfectly attuned or you feel endangered, as you have in the past.

MARK: It does feel like I've been here before.

ANGELA: I can relate to that. We can't redo the past.

THERAPIST: As you each get a better understanding of the other's needs, you may find that you become increasingly able to be responsive to one another.

Managing Disruptions in the Selfobject Transferences

While family members look to one another to fulfill selfobject needs, they also begin to expect the therapist to function as a selfobject. The therapist's failures in empathic understanding and responsiveness, or empathy with another family member, may trigger reactions that disrupt the treatment and require immediate repair for the work to continue. At the same time, these lapses foster therapeutic change if they are remedied sensitively. The therapist's ability to non-defensively examine and acknowledge his or her own empathic failure with the couple or family will usually restore the therapeutic alliance and promote the on-going work.

In this model, a major countertransference pitfall is the therapist's interpretation of what may appear as provocative behavior as a manifestation of resistance or primitive defenses. Instead, self psychological couple or family therapists must be sensitive to how they or others have disappointed, frustrated, or frightened the patients. It is crucial that the therapist understand that what appears as excessive demandingness, the need for constant affirmation, feelings of rejection and disillusionment, rages, outbursts, sullenness and withdrawal, non-involvement, glibness and superficiality, missed appointments, non-payment of fees, self-destructiveness and acting-out, and so on may be understandable reactions to actual failures in the therapist's attunement to or ability to meet selfobject needs, or to the anticipation and fear that such needs will not be met. This knowledge enables the therapist to refrain from reacting to patients in countertherapeutic ways. The need to empathically relate to the transference disruptions that occur inevitably in a self psychological treatment can be very taxing on, but ultimately rewarding to, the therapist.

MARK: I thought we were doing better but we had another awful row this week.

ANGELA: I'm very discouraged. I was feeling better toward Mark and now I don't know if we are going to make it. The day after we last saw you Mark told me to get out. I started packing and then he pleaded with me to stay. I have no where to go anyway so I stayed for now. I think we need to stop treatment for a while. We're not getting anywhere. Maybe we need to work it out on our own.

THERAPIST: You said that you were doing better. What do you think triggered the fight that you had?

ANGELA: I really don't know. We were both in a bad mood when we left here.

THERAPIST: I wonder if I did something last time to let either or both of you down?

MARK: Well, we talked about the session afterward and we thought you had been out of sorts.

THERAPIST: What did I do or say that bothered you?

ANGELA: You kept asking me questions about my childhood and my feelings. I didn't know what you wanted to know. You seemed very persistent. I thought you were intrusive and controlling.

THERAPIST: It seems as if you felt I wasn't respecting your privacy or going at your pace.

ANGELA: It seemed unlike you.

THERAPIST: I can understand that it made you feel as if I was insensitive.

ANGELA: Well, you were.

THERAPIST: I guess I didn't appreciate the impact that my questions would have on you.

MARK: I didn't feel you appreciated the progress I was making in controlling my anger. You didn't even seem to notice the efforts I had been making.

THERAPIST: You would have liked me to comment on how hard you have been trying and you felt let down that I didn't. Do you think there could be any connection between you both feeling upset with me and your fight?

ANGELA: I hadn't thought of that.

THERAPIST: Perhaps because you were feeling disappointed in and angry with me you both became vulnerable and needy.

ANGELA: That seems like a ridiculous reason to get into a brawl. Anyway, you are our therapist.

THERAPIST: You have both come to feel that I will be attuned to your needs, and when I did not seem to be that way the last time, it is understandable that you felt let down. It's been difficult for each of you to let yourselves trust that someone will be there for you.

Increasing Individual Self-Esteem and Cohesion

As part of couple or family treatment it may be possible to strengthen an individual's self-esteem and self-cohesion. This usually requires the development of a more intense selfobject transference to the therapist, who gradually helps the patient to acquire greater self structure through the process of optimal responsiveness and transmuting internalization, as discussed in Chapter 7. Individual sessions may accompany the conjoint treatment. For example, it seemed advisable for both Angela and Mark to do some individual work, and both wanted to see the couple therapist for this purpose. In Mark's case individual sessions centered on his fears of abandonment, low self-esteem, and lack of self-soothing mechanisms. With Angela the therapy dealt with her having been put in the role of a parentified child all of her early life, and on her fears of being swallowed up in a relationship and losing her identity.

ISSUES IN THE USE OF CONJOINT COUPLE OR FAMILY TREATMENT

Not all borderline couples and families can be seen together from the start. Sometimes such factors as the threat of potential violence, the rigidity of attitudes and defenses, volatility, scapegoating, paranoid and jealous reactions, and neediness may necessitate that family members be seen individually by either the same or different therapists. Despite the difficulties that inevitably arise from sharing the same therapist, it is preferable to try to use one rather than two or more therapists in working with a family since the problems of integration and collaboration are very complicated. One therapist is able to understand both the individual personalities and the family system and thereby work toward their shared goals. The use of the same therapist in these situations can work successfully if the individual family members can tolerate the problems that inevitably arise around issues of rivalry and confidentiality, for example, and if the therapist is able to maintain sufficient empathy for each family member.

Another common pattern is for one therapist to do both couple or family treatment along with the individual treatment of each family member from the start. This has the major advantage of permitting both individual and family work to go on simultaneously in complementary ways. Sometimes borderline couples are so afraid of being separated that they join in resisting individual sessions.

When a therapist starts with an individual patient the additional use of couple or family treatment conducted by the same therapist can be problematic but workable if the therapist is able to help the other partner or family members feel understood. The fact that the therapist knows the situation may be viewed as a potential benefit rather than a threat. Nevertheless, sometimes it is very important that one or both partners, for example, have his or her own therapist, with the couple or family treatment conducted by someone else.

While it safeguards the transference and does not pose conflicting demands on the therapist, the use of multiple therapists, each of whom sees different family members, is tricky because of the nature of splitting and the practical and interpersonal problems inherent in collaboration. Each therapist may be in possession of only some of the relevant data, and may develop countertransference reactions in which they become competitive with or regard the other therapist as incompetent. Close collaboration is important, although often difficult to maintain, in this type of approach. This model works well in in-patient settings, where staff can easily communicate with one another, enjoy good working relationships, and where the treatment structure is set up for the use of multiple therapists.

Some couple and family therapists favor a cotherapy model in which two therapists work together in sessions. This approach has several advantages. It helps the therapists to observe and intervene with difficult cases without getting as readily "sucked" into their pathological interactions, offers validation to each therapist, enables different alliances to be formed, and permits role modeling of good communication skills. Unfortunately, this is a difficult approach to work out from a practical and financial point of view, and requires attuned and collaborative teamwork. It works well in hospital settings when two therapists, each of whom is responsible for different family members, come together in conjoint family sessions. The structure already exists to make this model more feasible.

CONCLUSION

This chapter has discussed and illustrated the application of object-relations and self psychological perspectives to couple and family treatment. While it may be possible to integrate these two models to some degree, they differ with respect to their major principles and technical interventions. They both can be used either in conjunction with or instead of individual treatment, and are important therapeutic models in the contemporary treatment of borderline disorders.

References

Abelin, E. L. (1971). The role of the father in the separation–individuation process. In J. B. McDevitt & C. F. Settlage (Eds.), Separation–individuation: Essays in honor of Margaret S. Mahler (pp. 229–52). New York: International Universities Press.

Abend, S. M., Porder, M. S., & Willick, M. S. (1983). *Borderline patients: Psychoanalytic perspectives.* New York: International Universities Press.

Adler, G. (1985). *Borderline psychopathology and its treatment.* New York: Jason Aronson.

Adler, G., & Buie, D. H. (1979). Aloneness and borderline psychopathology: The possible relevance of child development issues. *International Journal of Psychoanalysis, 60,* 83–96.

Akiskal, H. S. (1981). Subaffective disorders: Dysthymic, cyclothymic and bipolar II disorders in the borderline realm. *Psychiatric Clinics of North America, 4,* 25–46.

Alexander, F., & French, T. M. (1946). *Psychoanalytic therapy.* New York: Ronald Press.

American Psychiatric Association. (1980). *Diagnostic and statistical manual of mental disorders* (3rd ed.). Washington, DC: Author.

American Psychiatric Association. (1987). *Diagnostic and statistical manual of mental disorders* (3rd ed., rev.). Washington, DC: Author.

Bacal, H. A. (1985). Optimal responsiveness and the therapeutic process. In A. Goldberg (Ed.), *Progress in self psychology* (Vol. 1, pp. 202–227). New York: Guilford Press.

Bauer, S. F., Goldstein, E. G., Haran, K., & Flye, B. (1980). The role of the hospital milieu in structural diagnosis. *Hospital and Community Psychiatry, 31,* 187–191.

Berger, P. A. (1987). Pharmacological treatment for borderline personality disorder. *Bulletin of the Menninger Clinic, 51,* 277–284.

Berkowitz, D., Shapiro, R., Zinner, J., & Shapiro, E. (1974). Concurrent family treatment of narcissistic disorders in adolescence. *International Journal of Psychoanalytic Psychotherapy, 3,* 379–396.

Blanck, G., & Blanck, R. (1974). *Ego psychology in theory and practice.* New York: Columbia University Press.

Blanck, R., & Blanck, G. (1977). The transference object and the real object. *International Journal of Psychoanalysis, 58,* 33–44.

Blanck, G., & Blanck, R. (1979). *Ego psychology II: Psychoanalytic developmental psychology.* New York: Columbia University Press.

Blanck, R. (1973). Countertransference in the treatment of the borderline patient. *Clinical Social Work Journal, 1,* 110–117.

Blos, P. (1975). The second individuation process of adolescence. In A. Esman (Ed.), *The psychology of adolescence: Essential readings* (pp. 156–177). New York: International Universities Press.

Blumenthal, R., Carr, A. C., & Goldstein, E. G. (1982). DSM-III and the structural diagnosis of borderline patients. *The Psychiatric Hospital, 13,* 142–48.

Boyer, L. B., & Giovacchini, P. L.(1967). *Psychoanalytic treatment of schizophrenic, borderline, and characterologic disorders.* New York: Jason Aronson.

Brandchaft, B. (1986). British object relations theory and psychotherapy. In A. Goldberg (Ed.), *Progress in Self Psychology* (Vol. 2., pp. 245–272). New York: Guilford Press.

Brandchaft, B., & Stolorow, R. D. (1984a). The borderline concept: Pathological character or iatrogenic myth? In J. Lichtenberg, M. Bornstein, & D. Silver (Eds.), *Empathy II* (pp. 333–358). Hillsdale, NJ: The Analytic Press.

Brandchaft, B., & Stolorow, R. D. (1984b). A current perspective on difficult patients. In P. E. Stepansky & A. Goldsberg (Eds.), *Kohut's legacy: Contributions to self psychology* (pp. 117–134). Hillsdale, NJ: The Analytic Press.

Buie, D. H., & Adler, G. (1982). The definitive treatment of the borderline personality. *International Journal of Psychoanalytic Psychotherapy, 9,* 51–87.

Bychowski, G. (1953). The problem of latent psychosis. *Journal of the American Psychoanalytic Association, 4,* 482–503.

Chatham, P. (1985). *Treatment of borderline personality.* New York: Jason Aronson.

Chessick, R. (1977). *Intensive psychotherapy of the borderline patient.* New York: Jason Aronson.

Chestang, L. (1972). Character development in a hostile environment. In M. Bloom (Ed.), *Life span development: Bases for preventive and interventive helping* (pp. 40–50). New York: Macmillan, 1980.

Comas-Diaz, L., & Minrath, M. (1985). Psychotherapy with ethnic minority borderline clients. *Psychotherapy, 22,* 418–426.

Deutsch, H. (1942). Some forms of emotional disturbance and their relationship to schizophrenia. *Psychoanalytic Quarterly, 11,* 301–321.

Druck, A. (1989). *Four therapeutic approaches to the borderline patient.* New York: Jason Aronson.

Eagle, M. (1984). *Recent developments in psychoanalysis.* New York: McGraw-Hill.

Edward, J. (1976). The therapist as a catalyst in promoting separation-individuation. *The Clinical Social Work Journal, 4,* 172–186.

Edward, J., Ruskin, N., & Turrini, P. (1981). *Separation-individuation: Theory and practice.* New York: Gardner Press.

Eissler, K. (1953). The effects of the structure of the ego on psychoanalytic technique. *Journal of the American Psychoanalytic Association, 1,* 104–143.

Elson, M. (1986). *Self psychology in clinical social work.* New York: Norton.

Fairbairn, W. R. D. (1952). *Psychoanalytic studies of personality.* London: Tavistock.

Fairbairn, W. R. D. (1954). *An object relations theory of the personality.* New York: Basic Books.

Federn, P. (1947). Principles of psychotherapy in latent schizophrenia. *American Journal of Psychotherapy, 1,* 129–139.

Fraiberg, S. (1969). Libidinal object constancy and mental representation. *Psychoanalytic Study of the Child, 24,* 48–70.

Friedman, H. (1975). Some problems of inpatient management with borderline patients. *American Journal of Psychiatry, 126,* 47–52.

Frosch, J. (1960). Psychotic character. *Journal of the American Psychoanalytic Association, 8,* 554–551.

Gabbard, G. O. (1989). Splitting in hospital treatment. *American Journal of Psychiatry, 146,* 444–451.

Giovacchini, P. (1979). *Treatment of primitive mental states.* New York: Jason Aronson.

Glassman, M. (1988). Kernberg and Kohut: A test of competing psychoanalytic models of narcissism. *Journal of the American Psychoanalytic Association, 36,* 597–625.

Goldstein, E. G. (1979). The influence of parental attitudes on psychiatric treatment outcome. *Social Casework: The Journal of Contemporary Social Work, 60,* 350–359.

Goldstein, E. G. (March, 1981a). The family characteristics of borderline patients. Unpublished paper presented as part of a panel, *Developmental deficits in adolescence.* 58th Annual Meeting of the American Orthopsychiatric Association. New York.

Goldstein, E. G. (1981b). Promoting competence in families of psychiatric patients. In A. Maluccio (Ed.), *Building competence in clients: A new/old approach to social work intervention* (pp. 317–342). New York: The Free Press.

Goldstein, E. G. (1983). Clinical and ecological approaches to the borderline client. *Social Casework: The Journal of Contemporary Social Work, 64,* 353–362.

Goldstein, E. G. (1984). *Ego psychology and social work practice.* New York: The Free Press.

Greenberg, J. R., & Mitchell, S. A. (1983). *Object relations in psychoanalytic theory.* Cambridge, MA: Harvard University Press.

Greenson, R. R. (1967). *The technique and practice of psychoanalysis* (Vol. I). New York: International Universities Press.

Grinker, R. R., Werble, B., & Drye, R. (1968). *The borderline syndrome.* New York: Basic Books.

Gunderson, J. G. (1984). *Borderline personality disorder.* Washington, DC: American Psychiatric Press.

Gunderson, J. G. (1987). Interfaces between psychoanalytic and empirical studies of borderline personality. In J. S. Grotstein, M. F. Solomon, & J. A. Lang (Eds.), *The borderline patient.* (Vol. 1, pp. 37–60). Hillsdale, NJ: The Analytic Press.

Gunderson, J. G., Kerr, J., & Englund, D. W. (1980). The families of borderlines:

A comparative study. *Archives of General Psychiatry, 37,* 27–33.

Gunderson, J. G., & Kolb, J. E. (1978). Discriminating features of borderline patients. *American Journal of Psychiatry, 135,* 792–796.

Gunderson, J. G., Kolb, J. E., & Austin, V. (1981). The diagnostic interview for borderline patients. *American Journal of Psychiatry,* 138, 1257–1264.

Gunderson, J. G., & Singer, M.T. (1975). Defining borderline patients: An overview. *American Journal of Psychiatry, 132,* 1–10.

Guntrip, H. (1961). *Personality structure and human interaction.* New York: International Universities Press.

Guntrip, H. (1969). *Schizoid phenomena, object relations, and the self.* New York: International Universities Press.

Guntrip, H. (1973). *Psychoanalytic theory, therapy, and the self.* New York: Basic Books (Harper Torchbooks).

Herman, J. L., Perry, J. C., & van der Kolk, B. (1989). Childhood trauma in borderline personality disorder. *American Journal of Psychiatry, 146,* 490–495.

Hoch, P. H., & Polatin, P. (1949). Pseudoneurotic forms of schizophrenia. *Psychoanalytic Quarterly, 23,* 248–76.

Hodis, L. (1986). The borderline patient: Theoretical and treatment considerations from a developmental approach. *Clinical Social Work Journal, 14,* 66–78.

Kernberg, O. F. (1967). Borderline personality organization. *Journal of the American Psychoanalytic Association, 15,* 641–85.

Kernberg, O. F. (1975). *Borderline conditions and pathological narcissism.* New York: Jason Aronson.

Kernberg, O. F. (1976). *Object relations theory and clinical psychoanalysis.* New York: Jason Aronson.

Kernberg, O. F. (1977). The structural diagnosis of borderline personality organization. In P. Hartocollis (Ed.), *Borderline personality disorders* (pp. 87–122). New York: The Analytic Press.

Kernberg, O. F. (1979). Psychoanalytic psychotherapy with borderline adolescents. In S. Feinstein & P. L. Giovacchini (Eds.), *Adolescent Psychiatry* (Vol. VII, pp. 294–321). Chicago: University of Chicago Press.

Kernberg, O. F. (1984). *Severe personality disorders.* New Haven: Yale University Press.

Kernberg, O. F. (1985). Melanie Klein. In H. I. Kaplan & B. Sadock (Eds.), *Comprehensive textbook of psychiatry* (4th ed., pp. 441–450). Baltimore: Williams & Wilkins.

Kernberg, O. F., Burstein, E., Coyne, L., Appelbaum, A., Horwitz, L., & Voth, H. (1972). Psychotherapy and psychoanalysis: Final report of the Menninger Foundation's psychotherapy research project. *Bulletin of the Menninger Clinic, 36,* 1–275.

Kernberg, O. F., Goldstein, E. G., Carr, A. C., Hunt, H. H., Bauer, S., & Blumenthal, R. (1981). Diagnosing borderline personality organization. *Journal of Nervous and Mental Disease, 169,* 225–31.

Kernberg, O. F., Selzer, M. A., Koenigsberg, H. W., Carr, A. C., & Appelbaum, A. H. (1989). *Psychodynamic psychotherapy of borderine patients.* New York: Basic Books.

Kety, S. S., Rosenthal, D., Wender, P. H., & Schulsinger, F. (1968). Mental illness in the biological and adoptive familes of adopted schizophrenics. In D.

Rosenthal & S. S. Kety (Eds.), *Transmission of schizophrenia* (pp. 345–362). Oxford: Pergamon Press.

Klein, D. F. (1977). Psychopharmacological treatment and delineation of borderline disorders. In P. Hartocollis (Ed.), *Borderline personality disorders* (pp. 365–384). New York: International Universities Press.

Klein, M. (1957). *Envy and gratitude.* New York: Basic Books.

Knight, R. P. (1953a). Borderline states. *The Bulletin of the Menninger Clinic, 17,* 1–12.

Knight, R. P. (1953b). Management and psychotherapy of the borderline schizophrenic patient. In R. P. Knight & C. R. Friedman (Eds.), *Psychoanalytic psychiatry and psychology* (pp. 110–122). New York: International Universities Press.

Kohut, H. (1959). Introspection, empathy, and psychoanalysis. *Journal of the American Psychoanalytic Association, 7,* 459–483.

Kohut, H. (1971). *The analysis of the self.* New York: International Universities Press.

Kohut, H. (1977). *The restoration of the self.* New York: International Universities Press.

Kohut, H. (1982). Introspection, empathy, and the semi-circle of mental health. *International Journal of Psychoanalysis, 63,* 395–407.

Kohut, H. (1984). *How does analysis cure?* Chicago: The University of Chicago Press.

Kohut, H., & Wolf, E. S. (1978). The disorders of the self and their treatment. *International Journal of Psychoanalysis, 59,* 413–425.

Kolb, J. E., & Gunderson, J. G. (1980). Diagnosing borderline patients with a semi-structured interview. *Archives of General Psychiatry, 37,* 37–41.

Kroll, J. (1988). *The challenge of the borderline patient.* New York: Norton.

Lachkar, J. (1985). Narcissistic/borderline couples: Theoretical implications for treatment. *Dynamic Psychotherapy, 3,* 109–125.

Lang, J.A.(1987). Two contrasting frames of reference for understanding borderline patients: Kernberg and Kohut. In J. S. Grotstein, M.F. Solomon, & J. A. Lang (Eds.), *The borderline patient* (Vol. 1, pp. 131–146). Hillsdale, New Jersey: The Analytic Press.

Lewis, L. A. (1984). The coming out process for lesbians: Integrating a stable identity. *Social Work, 29,* 464–469.

Lichtenberg, J. D. (1987). Some analogies between findings in infant research and clinical observations of adults, particularly patients with borderline and narcissistic personality disorders. In J. S. Grotstein, M. F. Solomon, & J. A. Lang (Eds.). *The borderline patient.* (Vol.1, pp. 107–130). Hillsdale, NJ: The Analytic Press.

Magdoff, J., & Greenberg, M. (December, 1988). *Self psychological treatment of borderline-narcissistic couples.* Paper presented at the American Association of Marital and Family Therapists Annual Meeting, New Orleans, LA.

Magid, B. (1984). Some contributions of self psychology to the treatment of borderline and schizophrenic patients. *Dynamic Psychotherapy, 2,* 101–111.

Mahler, M. S. (1968). *On human symbiosis and the vicissitudes of individuation.* New York: International Universities Press.

Mahler, M. S. (1971). A study of the separation–individuation process and its possible application to borderline phenomena in the psychoanalytic situation.

Psychoanalytic Study of the Child, 26, 403-24. New York/Chicago: Quadrangle Books.

Mahler, M. S., Pine, F., & Bergman, A. (1975). *The psychological birth of the human infant.* New York: Basic Books.

Masterson, J. F. (1972). *Treatment of the borderline adolescent.* New York: Wiley-Interscience.

Masterson, J. F. (1976). *Treatment of the borderline adult.* New York: Brunner-Mazel.

Masterson, J. F., & Rinsley, D. (1975). The borderline syndrome: The role of the mother in the genesis and psychic structure of the borderline personality. *International Journal of Psychoanalysis, 56,* 163-77.

Meissner, W. W. (1988). *Treatment of patients in the borderline spectrum.* New York: Jason Aronson.

Nurnberg, H. G., & Suh, R. (1978). Time-limited treatment of hospitalized borderline patients: Considerations. *Comprehensive Psychiatry, 19,* 419-431.

Ornstein, P. H., & Ornstein, A. (1985). Clinical understanding and explaining: The empathic vantage point. In A. Goldberg (Ed.), *Progress in self psychology* (Vol. 1, pp. 43-61). New York: Guilford Press.

Pack, A. (1987). The role of psychopharmacology in the treatment of borderline patients. In J. S. Grotstein, M.F. Solomon, & J.A. Lang (Eds.), *The borderline patient* (Vol. 2, pp. 177-186). Hillsdale, NJ: The Analytic Press.

Palombo, J. (1982). Critical review of the concept of the borderline child. *Clinical Social Work Journal, 10,* 246-64.

Palombo, J. (1983). Borderline conditions: A perspective from self psychology. *Cinical Social Work Journal, 4,* 323-37.

Palombo, J. (1987). Selfobject transference in the treatment of borderline neuro-cognitively impaired children. In J. S. Grotstein, M. F. Solomon, & J. A. Lang (Eds.), *The borderline patient* (Vol. 1, pp. 317-46). Hillsdale, NJ: The Analytic Press.

Piaget, J. (1937). *The construction of reality of the child.* New York: Basic Books, 1954.

Pine, F. (1985). *Developmental theory and clinical process.* New Haven: Yale University Press.

Pine, F. (1988). The four psychologies of psychoanalysis and their place in clinical work. *Journal of the American Psychoanalytic Association, 36,* pp. 571-596.

Racker, H. (1957). The meaning and uses of countertransference. *Psychoanalytic Quarterly, 26,* 303-357.

Rapaport, D., Gill, M. M., & Schafer, R. (1945-46). *Diagnostic psychological testing* (2 Vols.) Chicago: Year Book.

Reiser, D. E., & Levenson, H. (1984). Abuses of the borderline diagnosis: A clinical problem with teaching opportunities. In R. Fine (Ed.), *Current and historical perspectives on the borderline patient.* New York: Brunner/Mazel.

Sandler, J., & Rosenblatt, B. (1962). The concept of the representational world. *Psychoanalytic Study of the Child, 17,* 128-45.

Scharff, D. E., & Scharff, J. S. (1987). *Object relations family therapy.* Northvale, NJ: Jason Aronson.

Schmideberg, M. (1947). The treatment of psychopaths and borderline patients. *American Journal of Psychotherapy, 1,* 45-55.

Schwartzman, G. (1984). Narcissistic transferences: Implications for the treatment of couples. *Dynamic Psychotherapy, 2,* 5-14.

Schwoeri, L., & Schwoeri, F. (1981). Family therapy of borderline patients: Diagnostic and treatment issues. *International Journal of Family Psychiatry, 2,* 237-251.

Schwoeri, L., & Schwoeri, F. (1982). Interactional and intrapsychic dynamics in a family with a borderline patient. *Psychotherapy Theory, Research, and Practice, 19,* 198-204.

Segal, H. (1964). *Introduction to the work of Melanie Klein.* New York: Basic Books (Harper Torchbooks).

Seinfeld, J. (1990). *The bad object: Handling the negative therapeutic reaction in psychotherapy.* Northvale, NJ: Jason Aronson.

Shane, M. (1977). A rationale for teaching analytic technique based on a developmental orientation and approach. *International Journal of Psychoanalysis, 58,* 95 – 108.

Shapiro, E. R., Zinner, J., Shapiro, R. L., & Berkowitz, D. (1975). The influence of family experience on borderline personality development. *International Review of Psychoanalysis, 2,* 399-411.

Shapiro, E. R., Shapiro, R. L., Zinner, J., & Berkowitz, D. (1977). The borderline ego and the working alliance: Implications for family and individual treatment. *International Journal of Psychoanalysis, 58,* 77-87.

Siegel, J. (in press). Analysis of projective identification: An object relations approach to marital treatment. *Clinical Social Work Journal.*

Singer, M. T. (1977). The borderline diagnosis and psychological tests: Review and research. In P. Hartocollis (Ed.), *Borderline personality disorders* (pp. 193-212). New York: The Analytic Press.

Slipp, S. (Ed.). (1988). *The technique and practice of object relations family therapy.* Northvale, NJ: Jason Aronson.

Solomon, M. F. (1989). *Narcissism and intimacy.* New York: W. W. Norton.

Solomon, M. F. (1985). Treatment of narcissistic and borderline disorders in marital therapy: Suggestions toward an enhanced therapeutic approach. *Clinical Social Work Journal, 13,* 141-156.

Stern, A. (1938). Psychoanalytic investigation of and therapy in a borderline group of neuroses. *Psychoanalytic Quarterly, 7,* 467-89.

Stern, D. N. (1985). *The interpersonal world of the infant.* New York: Basic Books.

Stewart, J. M. (1985). The treatment realtionship: Real or symbolic. *Clinical Social Work Journal, 13,* 171-181.

Stewart, R. H., Peters, T. C., Marsh, S., & Peters, M. J. (1975). An object relations approach with marital couples, families, and children. *Family Process, 14,* 161-172.

Stolorow, R. D., & Lachmann, F. M. (1980). *Psychoanalysis of developmental arrests.* New York: International Universities Press.

Stone, M. H. (1980). *The borderline syndrome.* New York: McGraw-Hill.

Stone, M. H. (1987a). Systems for defining a borderline case. In J. S. Grotstein, M. F. Solomon, & J. A. Lang (Eds.), *The borderline patient* (Vol. 1, pp. 13-36). Hillsdale, NJ: The Analytic Press.

Stone, M. H. (1987b). Constitution and temperament in borderline conditions: Biological and genetic explanatory formulations. In J. S. Grotstein, M. F. Solomon, & J. A. Lang (Eds.), *The borderline patient* (Vol. 1, pp. 253-88). Hillsdale, NJ: The Analytic Press.

Tolpin, M. (1971). On the beginnings of a cohesive self: An application of the concept of transmuting internalization to the study of the transitional object and signal anxiety. *Psychoanalytic Study of the Child, 26,* 316–52.

Tolpin, M. (1987). Injured self-cohesion: Developmental, clinical, and theoretical perspectives. In J. S. Grotstein, M. F. Solomon, & J. A. Lang (Eds.), *The borderline patient* (Vol. 1, pp. 233–50). Hillsdale, NJ: The Analytic Press.

Tolpin, M. (1986). The self and its selfobjects: A different baby. In A. Goldberg (Ed.), *Progress in self psychology* (Vol. 2, pp. 115–28). New York: The Guilford Press.

Tolpin, P. (1980). The borderline patient: Its make-up and analyzability. In A. Goldberg (Ed.), *Advances in Self Psychology* (pp. 299–316). New York: International Universities Press.

Waldinger, R. J., & Gunderson, J. G. (1987). *Effective psychotherapy with borderline patients.* New York: Macmillan.

Walsh, F. (1977). Family study 1976: 14 new borderline cases. In R. R. Grinker & B. Werble (Eds.), *The borderline patient* (pp. 158–177). New York: Jason Aronson.

Wells, M., & Glickauf-Hughes, C. (1986). Techniques to develop object constancy with borderline clients. *Psychotherapy, 23,* 460–468.

Wheeler, B. K., & Walton, E. (1987). Personality disturbances of adult incest victims. *Social Casework: The Journal of Contemporary Social Work, 68,* 597–602.

White, M. T. (1984). Discussion of G. Schwartzman's "Narcissistic transferences: Implications for the treatment of couples." *Dynamic Psychotherapy, 2,* 15–17.

White, M. T., & Weiner, M. B. (1986). *The theory and practice of self psychology.* New York: Brunner-Mazel.

Winnicott, D. W. (1958). The capacity to be alone. In D. W. Winnicott (Ed.), *The maturational processes and the facilitating environment* (pp. 29–36). New York: International Universities Press, 1965.

Winnicott, D.W. (1949). Hate in the countertransference. *International Journal of Psychoanalysis, 30,* 69–75.

Winnicott, D. W. (1953). Transitional objects and transitional phenomena. In *Collected papers* (pp. 229–42). London: Tavistock, 1958.

Winnicott, D. W. (1960). Ego distortion in terms of the true and false self. In D. W. Winnicott (Ed.), *The maturational processes and the facilitating environment* (pp. 140–152). New York: International Universities Press, 1965.

Wolberg, A. R. (1982). *Psychoanalytic psychotherapy of the borderline patient.* New York: Thieme-Stratton.

Wolf, E. S. (1988). *Treating the self: Elements of clinical self psychology.* New York: Guilford Press.

Zetzel, E. (1971). A developmental approach to the borderline patient. *American Journal of Psychiatry, 127,* 867–71.

Zilboorg, G. (1941). Ambulatory schizophrenia. *Psychiatry, 4,* 149-55.

Zinner, J., & Shapiro, E. R. (1975). Splitting in the families of borderline adolescents. In J. Mack (Ed.), *Borderline states in psychiatry* (pp. 103–122). New York: Grune & Stratton.

Zinner, J., & Shapiro, R. L. (1972). Projective identification as a mode of perception and behavior in the families of borderline adolescents. *International Journal of Psychoanalysis, 53,* 523–529.

Index